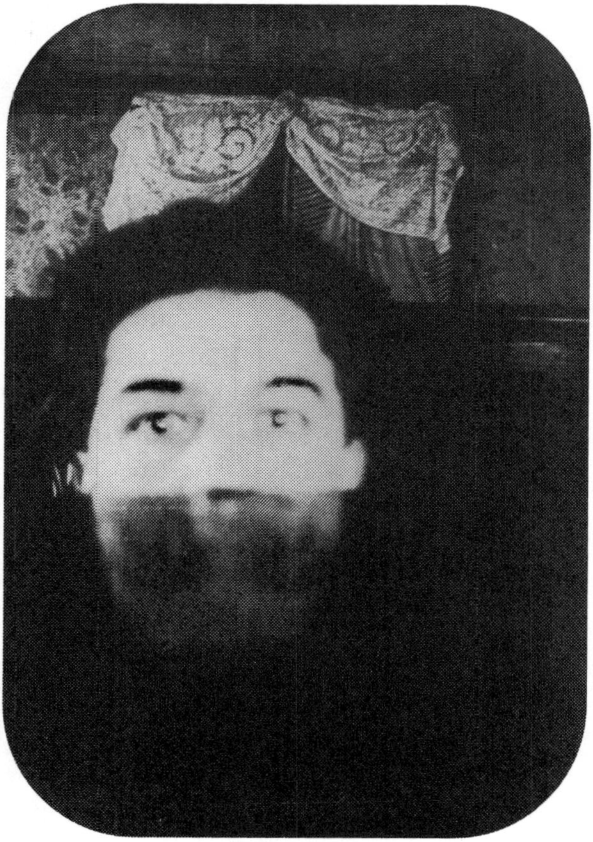

Bitter Blue

Tranquillizers, Creativity, Breakdown

BY THE SAME AUTHOR
(published by Peter Owen)

Fiction

Inhabiting Shadows
Isidore (Lautréamont)
When the Whip Comes Down (Marquis de Sade)
Diamond Nebula
Chasing Black Rainbows (Artaud)
Red Hot Lipstick (stories)

Non-Fiction

Madness – The Price of Poetry
Lipstick, Sex and Poetry (autobiography)
Delirium: An Interpretation of Rimbaud

Poetry

Black Sugar: Trisexual Poems

Jeremy Reed

BITTER BLUE

Tranquillizers, Creativity, Breakdown

PETER OWEN
London & Chester Springs PA

PETER OWEN PUBLISHERS
73 Kenway Road London SW5 0RE
Peter Owen books are distributed in the USA by
Dufour Editions Inc. Chester Springs PA 19425–0007

First published in Great Britain 1995

ISBN 0–7206–0892–9

A catalogue record for this book is available from
the British Library

Printed and made in Great Britain by Biddles
of Guildford and King's Lynn

For Fanchon Fröhlich

A *Books Consulted* section will be found on pages 135–6

Preface

Methods of withdrawal vary according to the drug and the sensibility of the user. This book offers a highly personal and subjective response to a twelve-year benzodiazepine dependency. My method of withdrawal is not to be advocated for those who are not in direct contact with inner dialogue, and the symptoms described were complicated for me by the colouring of a heightened poetic imagination and the residue of a breakdown which preceded my coming off the drug. Everyone finds their own method, and the availability of NET, counselling, acupuncture, group therapy and psychiatric help are there for each individual to explore.

My book deals predominantly with the creative mind, touching on the lives of those writers who have devoted themselves to inner experimentation. Lou Reed's apprehension of 'drug masturbation' or recreational drugs is quite distinct from the committed explorations of imaginative potential realized in their writings by Anna Kavan, Jean Cocteau and Henri Michaux, to mention but three of the writers I discuss in my study. The eccentric, the obsessive, the angular, the rebellious and the unconventional are my inveterate preoccupations, and all come together here in their alienation from self and society. The big leap into psychic geography.

The autobiographical nature of much of my book entails some responsibility for involvement, and the biologically intuitive need to disengage from a habit implies a directional route for some and not others. I came off the use of liberally prescribed tranquillizers because I grew to be so ill on them. That journey out of chemical reliance involved the risk of temporary madness, and the corresponding ordeal I describe in these pages. It is one journey, my journey, not everyone's. I wanted to get off benzodiazepines by the quickest route, but it took two and a half years before my cravings, hallucinations and disturbance subsided; twelve years of living in a chemically altered state. Many people cannot withstand the violent panic attacks attendant on withdrawal and they are quickly driven back to the drug. For often such attacks are too terrible to endure. My pills were always blue. Bitter blue.

JEREMY REED

Bitter Blue

Tranquillizers, Creativity, Breakdown

1

1978. I take a long flip back to the torrid late summer of that year, a quantum leap in memory that finds me sitting in the passenger seat of a silver Lamborghini being driven very fast towards the coast. It's my doctor who is driving me, his eyes don't leave the road, but our speech pushes tangential interests to a common centre. The Valium I took earlier, firing the drug up with Jack Daniel's, has me dissociated, cut off from the immediate and dodging in and out of the autonomous images that stream through consciousness. Later on I'll steady these free associations and make them into a poem.

I have been on Valium for a number of years. My original reasons for taking them are already indistinct, but I keep a bottle of the 10-milligram tablets in my jacket whenever I go out. They are a psychological support, and I can renew my prescription by a simple telephone call. It's easy. Latent panic, the anticipation of events that cause disquiet, the prospect of meeting people with whom I experience a discord of sympathies, parental tensions, sleeplessness, all of these psychological issues can be tempered by taking a number of blue tablets. I have always hallucinated, or have I? There is no symbiotic relationship in my mind between the drug and my state of feelings. That will come later. The damage is not sufficient yet for me to make a correlation between the two, for the chemical marriage is still in the making.

The car eats up the country roads, a whitewashed pub flashes over my shoulder like a jerky film image. I am so far separated from reality I might be travelling in a parallel dimension. We shall be there in ten minutes, and the sea will be rushing beneath the house, pushing a leisurely surf to a hemmed statement across pebbles.

I'm being told there is a new drug on the market, or rather that there is something to help those who are already addicted to Valium, tranquillizer junkies who feel the necessity to make a shift of chemical in order to convince themselves that they are not dependent on it. I like my blue tablets, they are the colour of the sky, they make me feel I am swallowing little circles of high altitude. Blue has always been the colour with which I identify. It's the sea, the density of a mood, solitude, the colour evoked by Marc Almond's voice, it's a French poem and a concentrated head of cornflowers bunching in a white vase. Blue is the colour that stretches like a cat in one's mind.

'The new drug's less addictive than Valium' I'm being told by a doctor who is also a friend. The data he is giving me is issued by Wyeth Chemicals, as opposed to the pharmaceutical monolith Roche. 'It's less habit-forming,' he tells me. 'And addresses a wider spectrum of nervous disorders.' I believe that. The chemical life fascinates me, as do most states of altered consciousness, coming as it does through a tradition of decadent literature via the romanticism of street drugs given mythic proportions by rock musicians. An iconic drug pantheon springs to mind: Charles Baudelaire's emaciated features and sunken bug-eyes, Antonin Artaud's ravaged body, lighter than a stick insect, Billie Holiday's stash hidden in a stocking-top, the barbiturate haze surrounding Marilyn Monroe, the bad acid trips symptomatized by the likes of John Lennon and Jimi Hendrix, and less romantic in terms of pharmaceutical iconography, the involuntary tranquillizer addicts who may be hooked for decades.

'We'll experiment. If you take these, you won't need Valium. You can have them at any time.' I am told that there is inadequate research into side-effects, and that new drugs arrive without a working biography. They are given a trade name and introduced into the blood. Lorazepam 1 milligram. And of course they are blue.

Most addicts can't remember how or why it happened. There was something wrong, but it couldn't be properly named or specified. Emotional subtleties get translated into pathological diagnoses. Once that happens, and the drug serves as an additional screen between the user and his original symptoms, so connections with the cause get distorted or disappear. What happened ten minutes ago? Most of us can't remember, and ten years back we were a different person. The word anxiety comes to serve a dual purpose: it denotes unspecified fear as well as apprehension over being cut off from the drug. There is also the problem of monitoring symptoms that have arisen due to the chemical, and that may have become the primary source of anxiety to the user. It is only much later when the addict attempts to withdraw that the mind learns to distinguish between the profile of complexes which led to the drug being prescribed, and the chemically induced symptoms caused by benzodiazepines. And there is a fear of madness linked to this. Most people taking Ativan or Valium are phobic and nurture a private fear of insanity. And those who are taking tranquillizers undergo feelings of constant disquiet that have no basis in reality. Ativan magnifies street paranoia, and it instates in the subject an irrational fear of imminent catastrophe. That car may break into flames, physical collapse in the street is a possibility, and what if I were detained somewhere for an unpredicted time without a supply of the drug? The idea is like steps at the bad end of town which lead to a black canal. A lion sits by a mooring-rope. I can smell its fleas and the rancid stain of its urine.

There was no formality about the occasion. My doctor produced a supply from his bag before writing me out a prescription. I would try them, and compare the effects to Valium. I was so sensitive to the latter that I could feel almost to the exact second when the drug wore off, a sensitivity that was to be increased by my taking Ativan, which has a short-term effect on the nervous system. When the Valium left my system I could feel my chemistry grind to a halt like a lift zeroing at ground level. And lifts come to represent pathological symbols to the neurotic. They have an association with doctors, waiting-rooms, big business, and so often one has to travel vertically to a consultation.

I like speeding. I have always produced so much adrenalin that something was needed for me to slow the pace. Some days I would imagine my head was lit by jet fuel, and the inner blaze burnt me. Ativan, I was advised, would rectify the imbalance and help me feel less angular to the world. Most drug users don't want to enter time, they prefer to live in inner space. They subscribe to Jung's condition of the *puer aeternus*, or eternal youth, and are reluctant incarnations; those who fear the intolerable commitment to reality and who value their inner worlds over and above participation in the capitalist ethos. Freedom or money? For many people getting a job is an end to whatever idealism youth represented. Day-dreaming, artistic preference, a heightened or imaginative sensibility, fantasy projections, a certain liberality of leisure time, a whole formative psychic geography is expected to be abandoned in the interests of a material society. I was told by the headmaster of my school that the pursuit of poetry was a feminine occupation and would bring me to ruin. Men entered responsible careers. I did not have a practical future, so it was thought that tranquillizers would dispel my anxiety and instil in me a greater degree of conformity. 'No future for me/No future for you' the Sex Pistols were to sneer through a vocabulary of abrasive insult.

And what about the patient's first prescription? Doctors assess types rather than individuals, symptoms rather than the complex psychology that underlies stress. There is a fascination between doctor and patient, the latter's vulnerability seeking sanction in the medico as a provider of cures. And pills are like money. The addicted hoard them. When I was totally dependent, I kept Ativan in every pocket. I would sometimes go out with ninety tablets on me. My fear was that of running out of them. I smeared the substance on my palms when riding in the tube. It was my blue tattoo. If things got scary down there in the dark I would coat my tongue with granules. I was always in need. I weighed eight stone four in my jeans. Chemical users are part of another species, and chemicals are linked to space technology, the streamlined tablet finding its correlation in the slim, undernourished figure.

If you know about the inner world, and if you are sensitive to imbalance, you can tell addicts. Not just those on needled smack, high on coke, or stoned on pot and its derivatives, but those pushed back into themselves by tranquillizers. They are the inner ones, people undergoing a confused state of dissociation. To be out on sedation is to sit in the back of your mind and watch the world as if on a giant television screen. Nothing is real. There is always this division between oneself and direct involvement with reality. Drugs are a form of chemical graffiti, they represent a vocabulary of incoherent signs, pointers to something that may or may not exist in the head. Ativan blocks you in, you can play games on the inside and no one sees.

Interviewed for *Zigzag* magazine in 1977, Lou Reed spoke of his interests in 'drug masturbation'. Taking drugs is a form of auto-eroticism. External reference is unnecessary when you are hooked on your own solitude and the manipulative invasion of chemicals. Nothing can reach you, and yet there is the feeling of cheating on the world, being out of it, and correspondingly vulnerable and beyond help.

Benzodiazepines are used as anxiolytics and hypnotics. The one induces sleep and the other sedation when given in divided doses during the day. Both are prescribed for unnatural states of anxiety. But 'unnatural' implies an unwillingness to conform. People who accept the preconditions of life don't need tranquillizers. We are back to the old criterion: those who fit into life and those who don't. Capitalism presupposes lack of choice. It informs the individual that the system is superior. To advance means to comply with specific regulations, to live outside, which means being unnerved and made apprehensive by the risks encountered in going against the grain. If you don't fit in with the status quo, which for me has led to conflict with the nepotism of the poetry establishment, life will be made difficult.

'Doctor, I want a scrip for Valium' is also a way of saying 'I need protection from reality.' Phobic or anxious people often find that threat comes too close, and that people appear to break through the instinctive boundaries we keep between ourselves and others. When you are deep-seated in tranquillizer addiction, too much of everything encroaches. You feel ill most of the time, and paranoid images free-float. The addict encounters a screen between himself and reality. The experience of alienation goes unrealized most of the time, you rub with fish eyes against the aquarium glass and through it encounter humans.

In their literature on the prescribing of and withdrawal from benzodiazepines, Roche Pharmaceuticals define anxiety as 'the final common pathway for different intrapsychic and biochemical processes. It is essential to remember this for benzodiazepines will affect the final common pathway and thus in the immediate short term help many anxious patients, but have no effect on the cause of their anxiety. Indeed benzodiazepines may mask important signs and symptoms and ultimately make treatment more difficult'.

Most GPs lack the time and the psychological acumen to consider the cause behind a patient's symptomatic disquiet, a situation not helped by the fact that a lot of people find it difficult to articulate an inner geography. They are too frightened to train a zoom-lens on the interior. And the availability of cure for any pathological disturbance depends on articulate discussion. Only by finding a descriptive language approximate to the symptoms may we project in sympathetic discussion. The rest is chaos; it is like sitting in the waiting-room of a deserted railway station, the floors choked by nettles, the clock hands on the wall pointing indefinitely to three o'clock. You sit there and the psyche bursts into a pyramidal green flame.

First symptoms are the most important. The patient will soon forget them when the drug takes over. What happens after that is the translation of a source into complex effects produced by the drug. And certainly for me, benzodiazepines fuelled a propensity to hallucinate. There are so many simultaneous multi-dimensional planes of reality, and yet on a functional level we are cautioned if we stray from an accepted level of shared communication. But the hallucinated perception and autonomous stream of imagery employed in most major writing from Lautréamont onwards, and taking in Dada, surrealism and rock music, suggest the continuous awareness of an earthquake inner territory. Writing becomes imploded after 1850, the European psyche detonates and we are still living in the fall-out of that psychic cosmogony.

Drugs are a part of this cosmogony. They can suppress or induce hallucination. Coming off tranquillizers may involve being subjected to months of terrifying hallucination. What I saw was lions, bleeding heads, faces that looked like crash victims, and fire. Bodies in flame, a crackle of orange in the tree-tops, conflagrations in the streets, and most dramatically, water on fire. For three weeks I was surrounded by flames. I could hear and see fire. The Hampstead ponds sheeted with vertical fire. If I were engaged in conversation with a friend, yellow flame would come between us. I lived in a cold sweat of terror. I feared being put inside. Other people were going about their ordinary day while I was sitting outside the Hampstead Tea Rooms, red lions sleeping at my feet, and the roar of fire licking across a blue summer sky. It didn't seem possible to go on.

Doctors fight shy of the fact that withdrawal after a long dependency may induce psychotic phenomena. Hallucinations are not observable distinctions, so they are little discussed outside of psychiatric practice. And for the patient, whatever is happening on the inside can't be authenticated, hence the terror of isolation. People talk about the loneliness of withdrawal, the fact that the user can relate only to someone who has undergone a similar ordeal, or to a professional who specializes in drug problems, and this is the most distressing and yet understated of drug problems. 'Out of it, man' is an accurate statement. There is just the intense fear that one will never get back and that a psychotic state will stay permanent. And it can be useful in states of terror to introduce a time factor to suffering. My psychiatrist suggested timing the anxiety waves. If you clock up fifteen minutes as the duration of extreme discomfort, you can establish a holding-on period when the agonized condition returns. It is important to realize that visiting disturbance moves on, it is fluent rather than permanent, except in advanced psychotic states.

But let us return to observables. You can detect fear in someone, it may show in their eyes and face, but you can't see the cause. The latter is subjectified, it is part of the person's private mythology. As children we delight in hiding. Later on we learn that fear symptoms often hide from us, and we in turn attempt to conceal our distress from others. So there's a hiding process involved. Most of us never really deliver our symptoms. We talk around them, frightened that they'll break loose and rush like big cats for the kill. There's an element of mutual deception on the part of both doctor and patient right from the outset of a benzodiazepine treatment. The doctor may be searching to typify a set of symptoms with a particular drug, and the patient may feel comfortable conforming to the diagnosis rather than discussing the deeper anxieties at issue. And so the deception gets buried; the drug sees to that. Thereafter the user will go on misidentifying the nature of his anxiety.

Being on drugs is like making a long-distance telephone call to the world which doesn't connect. Tranquillizer habitués are snowed out. So many milligrams last for so many hours, then the need repeats itself. When the impulse comes to detox, a signal indicates that a break in the pattern is required. I began to feel psychophysically ill each time I took my quota of the drug, and that for me provided the instruction to withdraw. I was discovering my own poisoning by drug toxins. Another urgent symptom that pressed me to be free of the drug was my apprehension that there was someone constantly watching me when I was alone. I began to draw up a composite physiognomy of the invisible stranger. Sometimes I would see him collapsed in the hall or the street. The whole tranquillizer dystopia was closing in on me, eventually to get clear from which means reconnecting with emotions, concentrated feeling, the return of the repressed – the sudden desire to live again independent of being dulled and inhabiting intranormal reality. It's a long process, this coming back stage by stage to an intended clarity.

If I could step back in time, twelve or fifteen years, I would be inhabiting the thought processes of a stranger. The knowledge I have now isn't applicable to then. These two people can never meet except in the infrastructure of memory. I have got to let that person go, and perhaps users are intent on assassinating their psychological past. The sense of no time or unreal time that benzodiazepine addiction creates is connected with the sense of unreality that most addicts experience. That in turn is an unconscious form of subversion, another manifestation of unconformity. It also implies secrecy, a pact between oneself and the chemical.

Most benzodiazepine addicts, unless they first used the drug for kicks, were prescribed it for unspecified anxiety – a condition that may be expressed through feelings of inner disquiet, unease, palpitations, dropped heartbeats, a change in bowel function, tension headaches, periodic dizziness or the apprehension of nausea, a whole range of symptoms that appear unconnected with the root disturbance. Something menacing has got into the aquarium. Eye, nose, tail or fin, the intruder knows where to hide. It is an undercover agent, a shadow. The man going to work in the morning stops half-way down the street. He can't go on. He wants to walk backwards and dematerialize. Panic. Dry mouth, muscular tension in the diaphragm and legs, shallow breathing. He feels cracked by pressure. The straight road with its familiar houses is looping like a snake. His legs won't support his weight, and that's only the beginning of it. If he isn't attuned to the inner world with its corresponding symbolism, the only accountable self-diagnosis is madness. The vulnerability is the worst of it. Most men are afraid to conduct sensitive discourse with their feelings. The latter function is considered to be a woman's preoccupation. And exchange the male character in the street with a woman and we have a reciprocal apprehension of imminent madness.

Let us look at a correlative taken from the visual world of painting. Edvard Munch's *The Scream*. In Munch's painting, completed in 1893, the hairless, agonized figure crossing a bridge, mouth frozen in an oval rictus, hands supporting the head, one on either side, as though physically sustaining a mind that rocks on the edge of spiral vertigo, has turned away from the two men who leisurely take in the view of an intensified scarlet and yellow sunset. What is the underlying fear behind this concentrated agony, this dramatic seizure which involves embarrassment, the turning away so that the viewer confronts the volatile scream, while the figures in the background remain absorbed in the landscape?

It is the sufferer's containment here that is of importance. His experience remains desperately private. Panic-attack victims, most of whom are using cerebral depressants, fear being found out in public. Respite from the attack entails privacy, and chiefly an escape from faces in the street and the brutal insensitivity of those who move in fascinated by the unfortunate. The neurotic outsider is disowned by the collective who fear inner turbulence and the potent imagination. Subjectivity is the one function that can't be controlled, and as a consequence it poses the biggest threat to rationality.

At the time of painting *The Scream* Munch, on his own later admission, confessed to symptoms that imply breakdown. Alcohol seems to have been the only sedation he used for overstrung nerves. The figure depicted in *The Scream* is observably suffering from psychotic terror. The face is one that figuratively embodies madness. Individuals become receptors for universal as well as personal suffering. On the highest level we transform symptoms into art. But where the sensibility is not creative, fear becomes caged like a panther. Mouth full of smoke, hands shaking, distracted over endless cups of tea, the victim sits it out, walled in by sedation. When I took Ativan it often gave me the feeling of living inside a blue room, an insulated cell. 'Blue blue electric blue/ That's the colour of the room / Where I will live,' David Bowie sings in that loneliest of all avant-garde pop songs, the lyrically fragmented 'Sound and Vision'. A hundred years earlier Rimbaud had discovered that solitary encapsulation in the idea of a room at the bottom of a lake, and of nations and ships gathered in the sky.

In *Opium*, Jean Cocteau's lyrical evaluation of drug effects and rehabilitation processes, a book wonderfully devoid of psychological jargon, Cocteau talks of the effects of withdrawal on the organism, the autonomous hallucinations which are also a part of benzodiazepine withdrawal. 'I recommend the patient who has been deprived for eight days to bury his head in his arm, to glue his ear to that arm and wait. Catastrophe, riot, factories blowing up, armies in flight, flood – the ear can detect a whole apocalypse in the starry night of the human body.'

I have walked out in the morning, shattered by withdrawal symptoms, to see the Hampstead ponds on fire. Flames sheeting across the water, roaring in orange cones above the trees, and later in the day the road was on fire, and I sat with a friend outside Maison Bertaux in Soho and was convinced that fire-engines roaring down Shaftesbury Avenue were converging on me, for I was on fire too. The fire is inside and outside. To whom do you tell that? Benzodiazepines are supposed to be antipsychotic drugs, but in the course of withdrawal the individual often encounters psychotic hallucination. And the conflict is psychophysical. A psychological need for the drug continues in the absence of physical symptoms. The nerves feel for the drug even when the receptor sites have closed down. The craving for sugar or alcohol at such times is just one of the intolerable disorders that accompany discontinuation of the drug.

Anna Kavan, an inveterate heroin user, is one of the most imaginatively articulate of drug writers. Her imagery, which has all the dynamism and originality of Sylvia Plath's best poetry, perfectly describes the feeling of nowhere to go inside or outside and the corresponding sense of isolation that inner captivity entails:

> Up and down, and up and down I prowl, what's left of me after they've put the pieces together again, like the mangy leopard in a Panamanian zoo, or the figment of somebody else's imagination. It isn't day and it isn't night; there's nowhere to go and nothing to do. The empty corridor filled with a stuporous stagnancy, with a sinister undertone of PR, is like the gut of a long white fish that is beginning to stink slightly. (*My Soul in China*)

The inner feeling of unreality caused by drug dependence has most users feel dissociated enough to be 'the figment of somebody else's imagination'. Apprehensions of being unearthed or disconnected from reality are connected both with anxiety states and with benzodiazepine reliance. People on tranquillizers feel so permanently disorientated that it takes an objective eye to suggest that the drug is the cause of the illness and has become the illness. Taking chemicals kills off the body's production of endorphins. The latter are the body's regulators and naturally generated pain-killers. Tranquillizers interfere with that process, and the addict in attempting to withdraw finds himself in dangerously unfamiliar territory. The brain has ceased to produce endorphins, and the supply of artificial chemicals has been cut off. This is where the conflict heats up in an arena in which craving takes on animal ferocity, and need becomes a sustained inner shriek. Let us hear Kavan again: 'A prisoner in solitary confinement inside my head, I'm banging and banging away to attract attention; this although I'm perfectly well aware that no one will ever come, no one will ever take any notice.'

The person banging around in one's head is the confused captive. Unsure as to why the thing began, sedated by a period of accepting chemical imbalance, the user is unprepared for the panic attacks that will ensue. Pharmaceutical corporations and doctors know of these symptoms only at a remove, and patients are encouraged to continue with a dependency rather than risk the terrors of withdrawal.

What the patient wanted originally was removal from anxiety and to gain distance on inner threat. In the external world you can screen yourself with your hands and protect yourself physically against terror. The gesture of turning away from confrontation is one we all repeat. But when the fear comes from inside, there are no instinctive methods of self-defence. You feel crowded out, the unwelcome visitant has taken up a seat in the psyche and is resting leather boots on your last resistance. No hands placed over the eyes can dispel the image. You would have to get your hands inside consciousness to arrest disturbing psychic automata.

I want to get back to the notion of sighting image. The taking of any drug that induces altered states of consciousness presupposes a sensitivity to this function on the part of the user. This in turn is a form of creative discovery. Most of us live by missing out on what is happening intrinsically. As a materialistic species we have been indoctrinated with the belief that inner concerns are dangerous. A fixation with inner states is considered a condition of madness. The societal dictum is to externalize, to do rather than to be. Shamanic dismemberment, paying close attention to the interpretation of dreams and the directives issued by the psyche are dispensed with in the interests of the individual adopting a functional economic role. People using street drugs want to get high, which means they want to go somewhere else, travel in another dimension, drop out of a predictable reality and entertain discovery. Baudelaire said in the middle of the last century, and French poetry predates any awakening in English poetry for almost another century, that we need to sail in search of the new. 'Le voyage' is all about breaking known frontiers and sailing into the blue. Boredom implies repetition and a saturation in terms of what we already know. The world often appears like an arrangement of familiar film props, stage sets in which we have lost interest. We want to break through and operate on a third and fourth dimension, we want to employ sixth and seventh senses. We end up naming things because we can't get round them, and so obstructions become nominative. Drugs employ a different vocabulary, they ask in the same way that a poem or painting should, that we realize the distinction between ordinary and heightened perception. I want to know something that my boredom level had previously denied me, I need to break through to the other side.

In *The Myth of Analysis*, arguably the most important book written on archetypal psychology, James Hillman talks about psychic reality and of the quest to find the mythical within the image, and as importantly the impulse to realize the creative and to potentize that energy through psychic modification. What Hillman is saying about the creative here has a lot to do with the expectations and frustrations of drug users.

> Why must the person who lives largely in terms of the creative instinct be damned out of common humanity? And the reverse: why can't the common man change his heroically romantic nineteenth-century concept of genius, so charged with ambition and envy, and be done with this fantasy of the extraordinary personality? Has not each of us a genius; has not each genius a human soul? Could we not find a similar extraordinariness within ourselves in our relation to the creative instinct as we experience it? Even without artistic talent, even without the ego strength of great will, even without good fortune, at least one form of the creative is continuously open for each of us: psychological creativity. Soul making: we can engender soul.

The creative person turns to drugs because of the judgemental values of a capitalist society: nonconformism is associated with bad economy. The person in search of a hidden self often uses drugs to sight unrealized potential. This involves not so much a turning away as a turning towards inner truth, and what exists without the structured fabric of society. Drugs are rarely responsible for a person's creativity, in terms of artistic originality, but they may contribute to what Hillman and Keats before him called 'soul making'. That is, the reconstitution of psyche, and the sighting of imaginal landscapes. The process of taking drugs is a reflective rather than dynamic action. It is separate from the creative function where the emotional impulse is volatilized.

Getting off, and coming off. Both imply direction. The benzodiazepine addict starts out expecting to reach a place other than suffering. Drugs appear to denote travel. They are the equivalent of flight – cellular space travel. I swallow and get there, you look on and don't move. That is one way of seeing the process. Benzodiazepines bind to receptor sites in the brain, and so dependency is formed. There is a growing sense in the user that the drug can control what the person can't. The person's conception of the chemical expands in proportion to his or her vulnerability. You can get to feel that the drug will insulate you from most imagined and plausible catastrophes. Its programmed control seems infallible. Whatever the situation, taking the drug seems the right thing to do, it imposes a screen between inner and outer realities.

Living on any drug involves a reconciliatory discourse between the taker and the substance. There is a need, often imaginary, to convince the mind of the necessity of the drug. Pronounced anxiety symptoms may have grown dormant, but the mimetic properties of the chemical reprogram that anxiety. And in the process of withdrawal the addict anticipates the discomfort that may arise in the drug's absence. And withdrawal fantasies are invariably and obsessively morbid. The fantasy may entail the fear of madness associated with depersonalization, it may involve projected fantasies of fainting, asphyxia, being set on in the street, being sick in a large shop, and panic states that remove control from the individual. Most phobic states are there before benzodiazepines are prescribed, and become intensified during the period of dependency. And most long-term users of Ativan and Valium develop agoraphobic behaviour patterns. Feelings of nausea, irrational panic at being in a foreign precinct, and all the disquieting symbols of a private mythology which for me might be connected with the sight of a bloodstain in the road, or portentous hospital buildings framing a backdrop against the sky, or the potential violence that seems to attach itself to certain streets or yards, all these things are components built into the agoraphobic's morbid sensibility. We are told that Nietzsche's madness was precipitated by the sight of a horse being whipped into a state of collapse in the street. Baudelaire's neuroses were aggravated by the sight of tenements which reminded him of his own poverty. Rilke feared hospitals and died at home, propped up on his pillows in the Château de Muzot. Most neurotic people come to read something of their own fractured inner topography in their confrontation with the public arena, but agoraphobics are involuntarily threatened by all unfamiliar spaces. I had the impression that buildings were going to fall on me as I withdrew, or that I would find myself in a district telescoping into labyrinthine streets, and that I would never emerge from the maze. I would run round and round in decreasing circles and in the process lose my memory.

What is it in fear states that we are trying to know or reject? The intolerable is most often caused by a disharmony between inner and outer. In pathologized cosmography, one does not easily fit the other, and the disjunction is what we know as fear. If I encounter the blood-stain in the street as the distillation of an accident, I'm provoking an internal scar, a pathologized wound that alerts me to nausea. The taking of tranquillizers may arm me against the revulsion I feel at the encounter. They may also prevent my feeling nauseous after I have eaten, or sedate me during the course of travel, but for many people none of these situations is going to provoke adverse nervous symptoms.

There is a question of the fear of insanity in this, an abstract unqualified state that we feel, even though we may have no experiential basis of madness. Phobic people fear going mad. Panic attacks, for which benzodiazepines are commonly prescribed, as well as taking on the secondary role of producing the state, are fast, rapid in their projection of autonomous hallucination, but are short in duration. The sweating, difficulties in breathing which may result in hyperventilation, tempestuous palpitations, the feeling of imminent death, the amplified distinctions of sound, smell and hearing are all characteristics of accelerated inner vertigo and not insanity, although the experience may make one feel that anything beyond this degree of fear is synonymous with madness. A panic attack is like a thirty-minute encounter with a personalized dystopia. And without foreknowledge of it, we may consider madness in James Hillman's words to be 'a disorder of brain mechanisms and breakdown of control'. We are in trouble because it's a head thing. You can't get inside to put the thing right, in the way the surgeon can repair physiological dysfunctions. Chemical chaos isn't observable other than through physical manifestation, the voices, convulsions and muscle disorders that symptomatize acute inner disturbance. As I write this book each afternoon outside a café in South End Green, I am surrounded by psychiatric patients from the Royal Free Hospital. Their idiosyncrasies are many and diverse, from schizophrenic dialogue to psychotic withdrawal; there's the man who moves a sugar grain millimetre by millimetre across the table, manoeuvring the granule towards some complex configuration; and there is the one who seems to be acting out a radio play for voices, and another who drags by always carrying a leather shoe in his left hand, his jacket on the wrong way round and torn across the back for this purpose. There is the young woman on high white heels who screams in the street and obsessively repairs her long hair in shop windows. She walks to meet herself in a state of inveterate distraction. Perhaps she would be helped if she met up with the stranger who is herself. What would they say to each other? And would they exchange roles? The one walk into the other?

What I note is the caution with which people treat madness, as though it is psychologically contagious. People's defence mechanisms to screen themselves are invariably those of ridicule, avoidance or disparagement, followed by the self-congratulatory affirmation of their own apparent normality. And yet the true creative state is one of disintegration, even if this entails a controlled focus on disorder. People fear madness only a little less than they do Aids. The dread surrounding it is one of primitive retreat and aggression. And yet most drugs including alcohol cause altered states of consciousness, risked by the taker in the belief that the effects are short term. Madness is dreaded because its effects are thought to be long term and because it often involves a reversion to the primal, and to a society that has relegated the importance of the unconscious to an inferior night place; then the imagination and the chaotic imagination are thought to be subversive to a material ethos. Antonin Artaud sees it differently in his celebration of those who are different:

> And you, lucid madmen, consumptives, cancer-ridden, chronic meningitics, you are the misunderstood. There is a point in you that no doctor will ever understand and it is the point which, for me, saves you and makes you majestic, pure and marvellous: you are outside life, you are above life, you have pains which the ordinary man does not know, you go beyond the normal level and that is why men are against you, you are poisoning their quiet, you are the dissolvers of their stability. ('Opium et sécurité générale')

It is the idea of 'going beyond' that Artaud establishes, a notion common to all drug takers whether the chemical is prescribed or bought illicitly. We come back to the idea of seeing and obstructions. We live with the belief that we are using only partial consciousness, and that an expansion of mind would relocate areas that we know but have forgotten. Poetry often has this effect on people. In the divisive break in his poem 'Le voyage' Baudelaire stops to ask 'What did we see?' The drug may help to locate the aperture through which we see, not like the paparazzi's telescopic lens sees the topless movie star by her private pool, but in a kaleidoscopic rearrangement of images. What is seen and known inwardly may be described as a parallel universe and is the space towards which we gravitate as counterpoint to reality. We live with the apprehension of a world at the interior; a place we would visit if only we could get there. The place hints at the marvellous. The need to get there has the attraction of driving a car towards the coast, the blue line of the sea shows up in the sky, and then through trees, is lost again, and a little later becomes a reality. Isn't it the place where leopards sit in the trees, jewels grow out of flowers, and the dead rematerialize by the roadside?

Today the light punches my eyes. I can't believe this is natural sunlight transmitting the ultraviolet that characterizes the ecological imbalance of the age in which we live. I feel as though a spotlight is turned on inside my head, a brutally interrogative light that magnifies my feelings of dissociation and nausea. Turn the light up and I can imagine my head exploding, the detonation chasing fire out of my skull. At such times the figure I have come to call the antagonist is there – the injured man, the sick man, the body lying dead in the corridor on my return. The collapsed figure is a projection of my inner wound. Sometimes my mind is fissured with earthquake scissures, zigzags are slashed into the earth, terracotta pots smashed into fragments. Damaged nerves may find their symbolic equivalents in images of universal breakage and cataclysm.

Medical research suggests that people on tranquillizers may find themselves acting out of character. Shoplifting, acts of irrational violence, magnified paranoia and baby battering in the case of women are just some of the more mind-twisting aspects of long-term benzodiazepine use. It is important at such times that the person acting out of character should have a witness, an objective mind that can draw attention to the changeover, the schizoid split in which the user flips. Acts that take place out of psychological character are the more disturbing for their taking place independently of those brain sectors which normally modulate behaviour. What occurs is an impulsive blaze. A heat-flash in which involuntary overreach is directed at someone or something.

I know when the imbalance is there. The stationary car appears to roll forward, accelerates down the road, and yet I know it hasn't moved. Or I see myself speed up the hill in a series of rapid, jerkily uncoordinated zigzags. The imagined movement is sometimes loopy, a pattern of spirals. I know I am in trouble. There are red flashes in the air. The unpropitious images suggest a bad phase to come. There will be panic, and in terms of withdrawal, the need to assess how low the quota of the drug can fall. That bus seemed too far to the left. It was my dead father's face that looked out at the smoking fog. And aren't my thoughts visible in my head, circulating there like fish in an aquarium? I shall be found guilty for the black fish on show, and the red and white ones will hurry through like the formation of music. My pockets are loaded with blue granules, my throat is parched, but I'm going to sit it out. And most days there are the big cats with which to contend. They convene out of the wind and become the focus of my hallucinated seeing. They don't threaten. They are mostly lions, but tigers and panthers keep their company. It is the why of their being there that disturbs. How is it I have formed the association? I am outside a café surrounded by guardians. I wonder what the others see. Are they conscious only of the chestnut trees grouped round a square, the traffic, the arrival and departure of buses, and the black girl with pink hair who can be seen suddenly stooping to retrieve an earring which dazzles on the pavement?

My cats are too personalized to be a backdrop to anyone else's vision. If I mentioned their presence, I should be thought insane. Inner reality is by its images a commentary on psyche. The seer is the privileged initiate, so long as he can address the image and retrieve meaning from its content. Under stress, the mind appears bilateral, bilocated. Inner and outer dimensions interconnect. My lions are situated in a mental space that also incorporates the field in which the girl has momentarily paused, left knee forward, right higher by way of supporting her weight, to pick up a green crystal.

Artaud declares: 'And as for me, I participate in your ills, and I ask you: who dares measure the tranquillizer for you? In the name of what superior light, soul to soul, can they understand us, we who are at the very root of knowledge and of clarity? And this on account of our insistence, our persistence in suffering.'

Artaud has proved one of the most passionately eloquent advocates of a vision that comes into confrontation with society by way of its representing a different reality. Not madness, but the concern to give inner values precedence over material concepts. Experimenting with opium, and later on with peyote in the course of his South American travels, Artaud spent most of the last eleven years of his life in institutions like Rodez, a shaman whose vatic poetry raged against ideological rationalism and pharmacological psychiatry. Artaud, like Rimbaud before him, and his contemporaries in mysticism and hallucinated experiment, René Daumal and Roger Gilbert-Lecomte, was looking for the break – the way through to living consciously in imaginative space. The violence generated by Artaud's thought, his vehement autophobia, his megalomaniacal pedantry, his conviction that madness is authentic knowledge, make him into one of the most individually subversive of twentieth-century writers.

In my internalized state I saw William Blake urinate, and the arc of his urine turned into a rainbow, then by midstream to a flaming prism, and by the end to a display of chalcedonies, emeralds and rubies. I have seen that. And I have seen sunflowers break out of cracks in the pavement with blood on their crowns, and giraffes decamp from taxis. I have watched people autocombust like black sausages popping out of the fat. I am talking about inner seeing, and how the visual cells of the cortex transmitted these images.

Robert Desnos used to compose his poems in a state of self-automated trance, not automatic writing so much as the reception of interrelated image clusters. Images attract each other, a ricochet, a vibrancy is neurotransmitted within the field of creative tension. This experimental period of surrealism, in which Desnos was the foremost advocate of 'sleeping-fits', had the latter attempt at one experiment to kill Paul Eluard with a kitchen knife, and on another occasion to encourage the experimental group to hang themselves.

2

Today I feel so ill that ends don't seem possible. Even embarking on a sentence is like undertaking a long train journey. How to live through the next thought and the one after that, disquiet racing through the nerves. The encounter with time seems impossible when one is in a state of intolerable anguish. How will there ever be an afternoon? And will a night succeed that blue space? I am experiencing dissociation and the fear that if death occurs it will involve an uprooting for which I am not prepared. The child's fear of being abandoned somewhere in a foreign town becomes the adult terror of separation from life. Where shall I go, and who will be there to meet me?

Addiction and withdrawal involve a departure from perceived notions of reality. Perception alters, and the sensory responses one had come to take on trust are no longer operative. The heart rhythm surprises by its irregularity, dropped beats, missed beats, and alarmingly magnified tachycardia. There is a hypersensitivity to smell, touch, taste and sound, and the smallest pain seems the precursor to a major illness. The edges of seeing hurt. Hallucination is a country, by which I mean it's another way of seeing, it's an implosively autonomous sequence of surprise events which instate in the receiver the upended perception that we acknowledge in terms of dream imagery but fear as a day-conscious realization. We have become accustomed to separating night imagery from daytime consciousness. We treat our dreams as belonging to an oneiric province over which we have little control, and the unconscious informants supply us with signs as to what is happening in psyche. When the weird imagery starts showing up out of time and out of place, we're running hard and scared. It's another dimension that has asserted itself as an alternative reality. I didn't run out of the house when it was on fire. I sat in the mental flames and watched the inner holocaust generate yellow, red, orange and green detonations. And the convention of big cats which gathered round me, had they come into inner space to find refuge from their endangered natural environment?

Albert Hofmann in his writings on LSD has pointed to the need to consider the existence of diverse planes of reality and to dispense with the formulated equation of schizoid perception in which the self and world are separated. The dual concept of the subject contemplating matter and being the passive observer of objective reality has given rise not only to Western materialism, but has come progressively to dictate the structures of art and literature. The imaginative artist is as distinct from this ego-dominated relation with the world as the drug user is from rationally based intelligence. Hofmann writes in *The Drug User*:

> The experience of such a comprehensive reality is impeded in an environment rendered dead by human hands, such as is present in our great cities and industrial districts. Here the contrast between self and outer world becomes especially evident. Sensations of alienation, of loneliness, and of menace arise. It is these sensations that impress themselves on everyday consciousness in Western industrial society; they also take the upper hand everywhere that technological civilization extends itself, and they largely determine the production of modern art and literature.

Social realism, by which I mean the tendency to report on a world perceived only through objective reality, has of course become the populist mode of expression in everything from the media to the arts. But at the same time it is the most limited form of sensory exploration. It is only when we turn inwards, and correspondingly realize the world transformed through the sensitizing properties of the imagination, that unity is achieved. I become the thing in order to re-create it. The image speaks for that transformation. Neural alchemy is realized at the moment of creativity. And most of the disordered states of mind we consign to diagnostic names are readings of inner states that are not necessarily transferable through creative dynamism. Psychotic hallucination is the subject of art, even if the psychotic is prevented by lack of clarity from articulating the vision.

Going inwards, tracing consciousness back to its origins, working the spiral back through imploded galaxies is the poet's art, the mystic's and the physicist's. What is inside is subjectively unquantifiable. The sensitive imagination, as we may term it, reveals itself through images. Hillman releases this definition in *Healing Fictions*: 'When an image is realized – fully imagined as a living being other than myself – then it becomes a psychopompos, a guide with a soul having its own inherent limitation and necessity. It is this image and no other, so that the conceptual questions of moral pluralism and relativism fade in front of the actual engagement with the image.'

Engagement with the image is an autonomous process. I cannot preconceive what I shall think. The formation and deformation of images are invited by the receptive, apprehended and constellated by the artist, and pathologized by the insane. But imagination is discredited and devalued by Western capitalism with its emphasis on rapid time and fast action. The process of undermining the instructive image begins in childhood. We are reprimanded for day-dreaming, we are told all the time to do rather than be.

In my strung-out state anything can happen. One hallucination telescopes into another. I see the passenger aircraft circling for landing permission over Hampstead Heath somersault into flames. All day the sound of jet engines menaces. I see a port wing crumple into orange fire. If I look up at the distinct fuselage standing off in the clear air, something alerts me to vertigo. I am afraid of crashing to a corresponding depth in my mind. I could get things back into balance if I took the drug.

Desperation. The naked wire of existence. It is like asking one's doctor, 'How will you help me when I'm dead? Will you be there to prescribe for me? Who will take care of me?'

Benzodiazepine withdrawal may involve persecutory delusions. Psychotic phenomena, seizures or ataxia may occur in patients with a long-term dependency on high doses. Massively oversensitized after years of emotional blocking, the feelings are suddenly alive to minutiae of perception. The subject begins to re-evaluate his past and to assess negative aspects which were in part induced by the effects of the drug. The resultant urgency to account for lost time, and to animate a retrospective sterility, leads to the frustration that is such a pronounced symptom of withdrawal. 'Where has my life gone?' the addict asks. 'How can I have been out of it for so long? Who was I when I was living such an emotionally low-key existence?' The answers are provided by increased awareness, a greater alertness to involvement in the world, a sense of psychophysical renascence.

Paranoid delusions take on global proportions when the user undertakes to withdraw. Is a friend the recipient of news involving one's lover's betrayal? Did the fixed stare in the street directed by a stranger denote knowledge of one's guilt, poverty, frustration? And who was that half-remembered person lost again to the crowd? There is the notion that one's private world is now made public, and that people are picking up on the conceptualized images forming in the mind. Paranoia seems to imply a raid on one's intrinsic space, a telepathic vandalism of the mind. Someone has found the code to get inside. It's a worse violation than rape, for it destabilizes sanity. Once somebody has found the way in, they might never go away.

I have forgotten who I am today. Tranquillizers induce that sensation, and while they are safer than their barbiturate predecessors in terms of OD risk, they impose deep feelings of unreality in the taker. And if I am someone else, I lack the composite biography necessary to become that fiction. I am in the contextual crisis, no one. NOBODY. You can walk the length of the street, take a bus or train, and still own to no identity. This no one won't stop to speak but may consult shop windows and fruit displays, and move on. I have been him at the ends of afternoons, someone close to falling off the edge of the world.

When I see a frightened dog tied up outside a shop, apprehensive that its owner may not return, I am taken back to the beginnings of my apprehension, the childhood anxieties that were to escalate to long-term addiction. As a child I was terrified that my mother would desert me in some large store, and of finding myself wandering through the town unable to recollect my name, address or identity. I remember David Gascoyne telling me of an incident that was his first childhood precursor to madness. He found himself one day compelled to walk out of school and to wander the streets of the town, and when a party came out to look for him, he lacked all recall as to his name, place and school. Who am I? The person you imagine me to be.

When one is nervously ill, one walks around a lot. It is the natural release to inner confusion. Pursued on the inside, one makes for the open. One is in effect walking away, although there is nowhere to go. Think of their attempting to get a distance on their amplified neuroses: Poe, Rimbaud, Van Gogh, Munch, Strindberg, Rilke, and André Breton carrying a rose in his hand, walking the Paris streets, expectant of the one woman's face who would catch his eye and prove the intuitive recipient of his intended gift. The creative mind as it formulates obsessive images goes in search of a correlative beauty. The elusively beautiful face becomes the reason to create. I am working the poem towards its anonymous receiver. Words will occupy the place of the absent one. They will breathe within their own tension field. You could argue that a poem by Hart Crane needs Valium.

Who is here today? What's on the inside, and how, if at all, does it connect with externals? Do I want to make the extension, or shall I remain subjectified with my inner chaos? The psychotic is one who has evolved a body language for hallucination. Semantic somatics. And if you embody a poetics, you also become it. Isn't that my difficulty? It is always impossible to tell if poetry is the medicine or the poison. What does Breton say? 'Across the diversity of these inconceivable flowers over there, it is you over there changing whom I love in a red blouse, naked, in a grey blouse.'

It can be the conception of a death fantasy, dying in public, rather than in private, which can be at the root of panic. Most of us internalize an imaginary death space, a precinct that may be connected to childhood imagery, or to the elemental contact with a garden or white beach, a place that is solitary and in which we feel protected enough to let go. As we discovered in Munch's *The Scream*, the agonized panic victim needs to find inner retreat in order to stabilize. I can be myself only within myself.

Breton tells us in *L'amour fou*:

> If I want the world to change, if I even mean to consecrate part of my own life to its changing in its social aspect, it is not in the vain hope of returning to the time of these stories, but of course, in the hope of helping the time to come when they will no longer just be stories. Surprise must be discovered for itself, unconditionally. It exists only in the interweaving in a single object of the natural and the supernatural, in the emotion of holding the lyrebird even as it is felt to be slipping away. To see natural necessity opposing human or logical necessity, no longer to try desperately to reconcile them, to deny in love the persistence of falling in love, and, in life, the perfect continuity of the impossible and the possible – these are tantamount to acknowledging the loss of what I maintain is the only state of grace.

In a world governed by accountants and the unilateral materialism of the masses, Breton's voice speaks with an even greater urgency. It demands that we trust in the marvellous. When I turn the corner I may see a bird with square black wings, rose bushes the height of poplars, their scarlet flowers sitting in the air, and a wind-tunnel in which ten thousand Marilyn Monroes stand with white skirts lifting above their hips. This is the real as it is manifested through aleatory lyricism.

Blues. Downers. The blues project. Bitter blue.

In terms of neural poetry it begins with Hölderlin and Leopardi. The nerves become accountable for deconstruction, deconstitution. They become an illness, a recorder of profound inner states, they resonate with the premonition of breakdown and madness as we know it in the twentieth century. The Romantics manifested madness, although inner states continued to be objectified, and qualified by a relationship with the natural world. Hölderlin was given a primitive form of shock treatment, his mouth gagged during the treatment. Thomas De Quincey in his *Confessions of an English Opium Eater*, a work that runs parallel with Baudelaire's own writings about drugs, gave authentic voice to inner terror, and his imaginary landscapes anticipate Rimbaud's *Illuminations*. Blues are there, not as yet as music but as a feeling of profound sadness. Wordsworth's 'We poets in our youth begin in gladness; / But thereof comes in the end despondency and madness' is never developed in his own work in terms of the imaginal and psychotic. In English poetry it is the outsiders William Blake, John Clare and Christopher Smart who give voice to the world of chaos and mental disorder. Clare seeks to find an empathetic solace in the natural world, Smart prostrates himself naked in the rain and invokes visionary fire, and Blake devises an elaborate symbolism to embody inner states. It is not until the French writers Gérard de Nerval, Lautréamont and Rimbaud that madness becomes the subjective quality of writing rather than the adjunct modified by allegorical or descriptive modes of expression. In Lautréamont and Rimbaud madness loses its association with social embarrassment and becomes a cause for celebration. It is the bourgeoisie who are constrained by sanity. Surrealism maintains the conviction that the normal man is the subject of ridicule, and it is only in the post-1945 world that the bureaucrat regains an inexorable hold on the arts. Safety has always been the enemy of imaginative creativity, the regulator that allows capitalist amateurs to manipulate the arts as a corporate body. Look at the men who represent the arts, they are invariably vapid bureaucrats, people dominated by ego and not psyche. Their power is political, it lies in the attempt to repress the indomitable fertility of the unconscious. Wars are fought to kill the imagination.

Ironically tranquillizers are prescribed for the hyperactive, the neurotic sensibility, the individual who encounters reality as a threat or has an over-abundant imagination. Sedation is used as a means of uniforming how we perceive the world through the senses. A whole populace has learnt to live by chemical restraint, the drug blocking access to the emotions by day, or sealing off oneiric vision during the night. Rilke finds voice for this in *The Notebook of Malte Laurids Brigge*:

The existence of the horrible in every atom of air. You breathe it in as something transparent; but inside you it condenses, hardens, takes on pointed geometric shapes between your organs; for all the torments and agonies suffered on scaffolds, in torture-chambers, madhouses, operating theatres, under bridges in late autumn: all this has a stubborn permanence, all this endures in itself and, jealous of everything that is, clings to its own dreadful reality.

Phobic obsession has about it what Rilke calls a 'stubborn permanence', a complex that threatens by its unmediated obtrusiveness. Phobias recycle themselves through the permeable or creative sensibility. My lions would not go away, nor would the projected vision of a wounded man lying prostrate on the carpet in my flat. But there is a subtle distinction between the creative and phobic sensibilities. The creator is most often he who adopts states, goes beyond empathy and realizes the fantasy, embodies it within experience, while having a defence mechanism that allows for detachment from the image after it has been creatively employed. The person who is neurotically distressed usually can't get any remove from the fixation; it acts as a gravitational field, and the obsession isn't transferable into creative expression. There are those who live out Munch's *The Scream* in mad wards and in the street.

What did I see the other afternoon, and where was the division between hallucination and reality? I saw a head open like a gashed strawberry, a man suddenly turned into a manic dervish, and a woman walking down the street clapping her arms above her head. She proclaimed that she had seen everything, that the promised land was round the next street corner. The way there was through a wall, a garden full of sunflowers, and then entry was achieved through admission into a big black pupilled eye. The eye swallowed some and rejected others. There was desperation in the faces of those who had to return. They came back to the street unchanged, and walked away.

This afternoon in Belsize Village I encountered a man frozen into what looked like temporary lupus, his posture was so stylized, so concentrated and contracted into intense dramatic gesture that he could have been taken for an actor engaged in extreme character portrayal. A glossolalia of obscene invective issued from his averted head, directed to the right. Somewhere in his mental line of vision he had met with an image so protean, powerful, shape-lifting that his consciousness was both attracting and repelling the inner fear. It was a deadlock combat. Traffic ticked its way through Buckland Crescent, customers selected flowers, vegetables and fruit from the greengrocer's, pedestrians went about their day, but this man was focused into another more powerful vision. He might have been the victim of invisible assassins, a closing circle of maniacal terrorists. He wasn't going to unlock until the issue was resolved, the fixation freed to be replaced by another. If this man could have articulated his vision with lucidity, delivered it with poetic crystallization, we might have been still nearer to learning of the multidimensional universes located by altered states of mind, whether induced by imaginative vision, psychotic hallucination or hallucinogenic substances like LSD and mescalin derivatives. In 'Le poème haschisch', Baudelaire draws a distinction between natural and induced hallucination:

> There is an important difference between the pure hallucination, which doctors often have the opportunity to study, and hallucination which involves an error of the senses, in the mental state induced by hashish. In the first case, the hallucination is sudden, perfect, and inevitable; in addition, it finds neither pretext nor excuse in the world of external objects. The patient sees shapes or hears sounds where none exist. In the second case, the hallucination is progressive, nearly voluntary, and doesn't become perfect; it materializes only in the imagination. . . . The disordered vision of the man on hashish sees strange shapes, which are a deviation from the normal. The energy, the reality of the hallucination in no way invalidates the original distinction. One kind has its origins in the immediate, the other does not.

Natural or autonomous hallucination is in Baudelaire's terms the more authentic revelation. It involves direct seeing by surprise.

What registers hasn't been invited, and is the more electrifyingly disturbing for that. Defences don't exist. I have seen people metamorphosed into animals in the street, a regiment double down the deserted road, men in battledress crashing towards a location situated in a parallel universe. I am unlikely to encounter these men again. If the hallucination recurred, I might be in trouble.

I have a friend who collapsed in the street after believing he had been shot by soldiers. Prostrate, screaming, he ended up inside, another temporary inhabitant of a psychiatric wing, the doctors intent only on repressing his tendency to hallucinate and blocking it in by drugs as a wrong way of seeing. What was this man's distress that drove him to a state of paranoid apocalypse? Where did the bullet register? In his head, his arm, his chest? The bullet penetrated, creating psychosomatic pain, and paralysed something in his nervous system. And now he would always remain someone who had been assassinated. He would live as one of the undead, the half-deaths who live on as psychotic simulacra. None of Francis Bacon's anamorphoses observe any other terror than their own, the nervous holocaust that has caused the face to split like meat along the bone is a private intensification, a one-to-one confrontation with inner catastrophe. The obscene faces that gather at the sight of an accident, or a man disintegrating into delirious raving on the pavement, are unprepossessed, they are a gesture of fascination with the victim, a compulsion to witness something within themselves which remains unrealized as a potential. But the subjective configuration could occur. This is the attraction. We all want release into states that we wouldn't naturally encounter, and in order to establish empathy with suffering we are compelled to witness how others respond to pain.

And so we return to the image of the wounded man. The breakdown figure. The one who is vulnerable. Feeling he suffers, suffering he is rejected by a materialist society, and finally guilty about his difference, he cracks.

To the person who has encountered breakdown, the gradations of progress back to any form of stability are fractionally slow. Advance is by millimetres; a bad letter, a rebuff, a psychological refutation are sufficient to blow one back. For me there was sometimes a big white bear freezing me in my head. What if it stepped out? And there was the man who walks face down in the cold, alienated when others are coming home from work in the evening and acutely aware of his difference. He takes his head back home and stands it on the table. If his body arrives it will be hours later. Where does he go the next day? A head plugged into fear. The local café, a street corner, the rift in the horizon where a headless community are a psychic and physical reality?

Go out in the afternoon, and one in every four people you pass has benzodiazepines in their chemistry. Cerebral depressants have become a way of life to a technocratic universe. And there is the psychological wind-tunnel that accelerates as we approach not so much a distinctive millennium as the despiritualized cosmic catastrophe. There is nowhere to go, so we all go with it. The mad have seen this always – a post-psychotic infinity, aeons imploding in receptor sites, civilizations burning out in maniacal collisions. The eye-witnesses of inner cataclysm are conveniently diagnosed mad, and drugs take care of the rest. The prophetic voice and the apprehension of the chaotically marvellous become a state to be cured by anti-convulsants. The wolf-man and lycanthropic consciousness are silenced.

I keep on monitoring sight as it happens independent of externals. It is on the inside that thought-traffic occurs, the big issues, the small ones, the surprises. It is a different mind one takes outdoors, there is a subtle distinction between sighting in a familiar room and conducting an inner dialogue in public. Private thinking is liberally subjectified, expansive as it arrives rather than being checked in its conceptualization, as occurs in the presence of others. We get caught out in public. People want to stem the inner stream of consciousness; they will admonish another's preoccupation and dispel it by intrusion. It is considered dangerous to go away, and to keep on travelling in that direction suggests an exclusion of reality, a preclusion of others. It is considered self-indulgent to go inwards. What you find there has no extraneous context. Breton:

I am walking on cork. How mad they must have been to stand a mirror in all this debris. And the taps spitting out steam! Supposing there are taps. I am looking for you. Even your voice has been taken away by the fog. The chill sends an emery board over my nails, ninety metres long (at a hundred I will have no nails left). I desire you. I desire only you. I caress the white bears without reaching you.

The white bears. I want to return to these. They too have waited in my nervous precinct, not as symbols of oneiric activity but as day-conscious intruders. Or was it I who advanced on their territory? They were part of white silence. They had blue eyes which never closed. Meeting them was an experience like walking through a mirror to confront the imagined. The big freeze, the big sleep. Go too far and the snow is barbiturate. Open your mouth and you overdose through crystals.

Tranquillizers are convenient in size, they are aesthetically right in proportion for the mouth, and more particularly the tongue. Perhaps this is a part of the problem: the ritual of oral fixation. Blue, white or green are colours that are psychologically palatable. The colour can be assimilated, added to the chemistry, it becomes a form of tonal modification of the nerves. Doctors don't usually connect with the fetish. To the user it is a ritual, a form of fellatio with the dissolving chemical. And after that the process of imagining what is happening with the assimilated substance, this too is a part of the fantasy. It is a non-medical hypothesization; drug users pick up medical knowledge, one has only to cite Burroughs's writings to realize that, but the process is still imagined, it is not biologically conceived. It lacks scientific sighting. Granules are binding to receptor sites in the brain, but most users either envisage the process abstractly or not at all. If you want to dull or kill yourself on drugs, the biochemical process is imaginary. It is like thinking of the bottom of the sea, of fish and fauna you have never seen. What is down there? Marine genocide. Hillman: 'We all have dispersed consciousness through all our body parts, wandering wombs; we are all hysterics. Authenticity is in the illusion, playing it, seeing through it from within as we play it, like an actor who sees through his mask and can only see in this way.'

The notion of dispersed consciousness, or the imaginative input living within the physical and growing to be the psychophysical, a holistic notation of being, is one little considered by doctors or biological psychiatrists, but as Hillman expresses it, 'We are all hysterics.' Dispersion is a part of stress, and the latter is necessary to creativity. The man writing poetry catches fire in each body zone, and release is an electric interaction between consciousness and nerves.

I have known psychotic hallucination, or the reverse side of reality. I have seen myself eviscerated, my mind blown out like unravelled tape across the room, images beating violently against the walls, and the fear that the state would not subside. Eagles spaded my intestines, my body fried in the dust. I was in danger of not getting back and staying there on the other side where the dialogue is so different, the visuals in continuous and disjunctive metamorphosis. I saw a salamander basking on a wall in the Finchley Road; my friend Ruby was standing in the middle of the traffic, reading out of a black book, and no collision occurred. Cars went through her to right and left without the squeal of brakes or a momentary relapse of speed. Ruby was inviolable by way of over-presence. And I have a friend called Rolf who sees fire boiling out of walls, and the incineration of his office colleagues as they sit at their desks. Their transformation is into death images, skeletons lying in open coffins. These are realities observed by someone going about a routine office day. What are we seeing at any given time? Most of us are intent on repressing the hidden image – it can't break through, so life acquires a uniformity of thought, a repeatedly modulated stream-of-day-consciousness. Rilke writes: 'I began to walk quietly as soon as I saw her. When poor people are thinking, they shouldn't be disturbed. Perhaps their idea will still occur to them.'

The idea crystallizes when its distinguishing properties separate it from flux. The poet's courage is one of actively engaging with disorder. He seeks to pull the tiger out of the flames by its tail. Using drugs may involve a similar but involuntary encounter with imagery, the risk involved by taking street drugs being one of a chemicalized raid on the unconscious, whereas the poet's journey to the interior generates a more organic stream of imagery.

But medicine is about cure, not differentiable visual associations. No doctor asks you what you 'see' when you take tranquillizers or any other pharmaceutical product. They might ask you what you feel in terms of side-effects, but usually knowledge provided with a prescribed drug is minimal. This is part of a doctor's professionalism, the hermetic investment in pharmaceutical knowledge that the patient presumes to be infallible. The drug must work, and if it doesn't, a second, third or fourth will be prescribed. The doctor knows what is going on, the patient hasn't a clue. The patient fantasizes over the opposition between illness and chemical, the imaginary combat between organic and synthetic.

We know that when Rilke was dying of pernicious leukaemia, he refused to have his illness named. Naming it would implant a definition quite distinct from his suffering. As long as he could internalize the idea of his illness, and attempt to reconcile it with a notion of mental cure, he could continue to keep the illness at a remove. His body rashed with black pustules, which ulcerated his mouth and throat, and unwilling to be seen by anyone except his nurse and a doctor, Rilke prepared for his psychic migration. The big spaces were pulling him out of his gravitational field. Rilke elected to die as someone whose death was still an expression of his work, an inner reverberation – the man sitting up on his pillows, meditating his way into death, the subject about which he had written so often. And was the reality approximate to his imagined expression of death? Was there anything or anyone there? Did he follow the tunnel until a luminous blip of light connected with him in the form of a guide? One should remember the opening line of the *Duino Elegies*: 'Who if I cried would hear me?' Was he heard in life or out of it? He had always worked against the grain, taking poetry to places so inward that no one had been there before. Rilke embodied the thing as it lives through identified animation, the inner state as it is known as a reality, and not as a pathologized symptom. Like Jung, Rilke identified with the inner as the vocabulary through which we know ourselves and the world. Going into the world often means an involvement in the over-known, a metaphoric statement about a statement. Rilke didn't need to comment on the known; he had already rejected it for the unknown. And this was an individual's far-reaching protest. Society has never liked insiders, nor do universities or a class-dominated literary establishment. And one way to warn people off the interior is of course to nullify the brain with tranquillizers. The individual who aspires to go inside, or become in Burroughs's terms 'a cosmonaut of inner space', suffers intolerable rejection. The man huddled into himself writing at a café table or the one screaming at passers-by on the pavement are both in interiorized situations with their own purchase on reality. They have each brought into the world a sensitivity that has resisted acclimatization to convention. To be different means to think independently of social systems.

And for those who break, doctors are there to supply demand, and the pharmaceutical companies offer them a commission. Two organizations that are non-users conspire to hook the individual who feels unable to cope with the distinction between inner and outer worlds. In breakdown states there is a feeling the image has come too close. There is not enough space between me and it to develop a qualitative differentiation, and so panic registers. Why am I being attacked from the inside? Why have customary defences collapsed? Inner perspective has become unbalanced. And what if my perception of the world never rights itself again? The huge catastrophes will go on burning. I shall autocombust as a consequence of nervous volatility. Waves of fear are like that, they peak and subside, peak and subside, and register as current in the muscles. It is like the electric flash, the charred brain cells of the protagonist in Robert Lowell's poem 'Florence'.

Hot and cold. Fear creates both. The alternation is part of nervous illness, part of withdrawal. Sweating is succeeded by spasm or shaking. Throat, chest and legs shiver, it is hard to stay upright on the earth's surface. My friend who collapsed in the street was taken to a chemist. Suspected of being on drugs he was denied any proper attention. His alleviant was a bottle of whisky purchased from the nearest supermarket. And to cradle a bottle in the High Street, draw on it desperately, could attract a policeman's eye, another vehicle of suspicion. You go from one state of alarm to another and nothing is explained, both states belonging to the nervous outlaw. The sexual outlaw is nocturnal, the nervous one belongs to day and night, and both are in danger of arrest, being extracted from a private space and exposed to public inquisition. The leather-jacketed cult in the woods behind Jack Straw's Castle are in search of Sado-masochistic revelation, a realization through pain inflicted or received that an inner dimension expands in accordance with orgasm. For the disturbed, the discourse is with hallucination or image. The unpropitiated symptom, which is in turn pathologically menacing, looks for transference to something referentially consoling.

A breakdown is a series of inner upheavals and chaotic disturbances that register in the psychophysical body. There is no easy way out of this dilemma: obsession attracts fear to its gravitational field. The insider lives as a social outsider. We are back to Rilke and his observation of Paris: 'People come here to live? I thought they came here to die.' These opening lines to *Malte Laurids Brigge* sound the existential pulse of the twentieth century and predate Sartre's *La nausée* by almost thirty years in their evocation of man's impossible dichotomy: the trauma of living and the insuperable fear of death. Both states are perceived as unacceptable. This is the pivotal despair of psychic visualization. Seeing implies going beyond, if we think of it in terms of the visionary. Getting rid of matter for anti-matter, transforming stones into gold, images into poetry. Blake's 'A robin redbreast in a cage/ Puts all Heaven in a rage' is simply the frustration of the unattainable. The bird knows it is in space, but it is confined by a cage. The poet knows he is in experience, but he is constrained by language.

Mental travel is a dangerous occupation in the material world. It can't be justified in quantitative terms. The doctor is on the right side of illness because his role is translatable into terms of money – the man who administers drugs receives money for his knowledge of how pharmaceuticals interact with the body's chemistry. The patient can't convert his individual dilemma of having crossed over into the unrealizable to similar gain. The world would have us know that there is something wrong about being mentally or nervously ill. Take away the romantic aura investing the deranged artist, and the fascination with the schizophrenic's open-ended dialogue, and the reality is very different. Someone has crashed barriers, and usually they don't know how they got there. The only way back is to report on images, dreams and the static that buzzes in the nerves like a precipitant storm.

In the latter part of the twentieth century we risk missignposting the way. The direction towards unmediated technocracy denies the real issues, those of accommodating the imagination to the themes of creativity, illness and death. Wrenched off the highway in a Ballardian collision of metal and glass, made obsolete by computerology, terrified in the face of the virologist's report, man is forced to go inner with his dream of an aquarian millennium. And death is not so much an alternative to life as the only space into which we can expand, in the way dimensions alter in sleep and dreams. At the end of the day we go somewhere else. We encounter dream reality. As a species we submit involuntarily to dying, and resist the earlier initiation into the process which the imagination should afford. Art is a preparation for dying, for it presents the inner topology which in time will become a reality. Where was I? Watching a hand balanced on a coral summit as it emerges from the sea. Walking in trance through a crystal forest. The abrupt switch is to a stag sitting on the bonnet of a red sport car. What I know are captions, fictions, speed flashes which recur. Neurosis or obsession is simply a crystallization of inner geography. The complex familiarizes the individual with realities that exist with the same intensity as detail in a Max Ernst painting. The discoveries in nervous illness are also the findings of art. The healthy individual is resistant to both; he is like the swimmer who never takes up scuba diving. He will never see further than his eye permits, or be aware of the subaqueous journey inside the whale's belly.

Those who are ill, live in a different time from those who are not. It is a precinct into which the possibilities of breakdown and death are admitted. They are its occasional visitors, potential occupants. And illness is a time of contemplative fantasy, and if the impairment is physical then the mental faculties compensate by developing an autonomous life. We go somewhere else awaiting recuperation.

And withdrawal. Today I have been out searching for a face, someone whose sympathies will accord with my own. It is a muted, pink, late September afternoon. The street becomes the terrifying arena in which one contests one's loneliness with the coming night. 'A hand, your hand then,' Robert Lowell wrote to Anne Adden in a poem called 'Mania', his overwired circuit looking for protection against the crash, the wrecked room, overturned bottles, the long drop into the dark. When Lowell came round, it was often in a hospital, strait-jacketed, chain-smoking to feed his rapacious nerves. A wall can take the shoulder, but a hand bunched in the warmth of fingers is an emotional pivot against loss of identity.

What are the choices when we elect to live in the fantasy conceptions of death? I want a way out, but the organism is still functional, the heart pushing blood through the arteries, the lungs regulating breath. But my mind is creating ends. I should like to be reviewing my mind from the vantage-point of death. I should like to live in the interaction between the two states, evaluate death while still having the alternative to live. Which state is preferable? In my death fantasy I have integrated psychic and physical characteristics which I don't do here. The aspiration to fearlessness in contrast to my nervous obsessions, and to permanent and perfect youth in contradistinction to growing older, are two preoccupations that feed this fantasy. The *puer aeternus* has scorched its wings. I must keep on acquainting myself with death in order to live. I shall become someone else by imagining the contrast. I shall be partially realized in this pink September dusk, the plane trees holding dominance in the High Street, no red leaf, just a fringe of yellowing in the green foliage.

The drug user never reintegrates with society. He measures his scar, the hairline fissure in the overall fabric, against the apparent unadventurousness of the collective. Bits are missing, so the pieces will never properly fit again. But there is an advantage here in the knowledge that more experience gets in as a consequence. There is an openness, a permeability that leads to collisions on the inside. The awareness that no one is ever safe, and that what we take on trust, the things that don't register consciously but which are going on all the time below the surface, are suddenly blindingly made clear as the meaning or contents of life. I find the idea of contents important. We spend a lot of time in absent thought, wishing neither to locate nor repel an image, and prepared to let everything go rather than look out to arrest a theme that jolts us back into time. In time, I need to be aware; in space, I can drift without fixed image points.

The history of twentieth-century poetry and art is also a narrative of breakdown. Survival is seen as all in the face of nervous catastrophe. Without even the knowledge of a global future, the poet faces the possibilities of suicide, non-readership, marginalization by the media and the prospects of carrying the unwanted into the unknown. 'Sucked screaming into old age and death', as John Ashbery puts it. Imaginative writing has become once again the prerogative of the underworld, those five hundred representatives of consciousness who have been the poet's public ever since Baudelaire and the beginnings of the modern sensibility. The only way forward is by infiltrators, carriers of the message who pass it on by word. I deliberately use the word 'carriers' with all its HIV death connotations in the nineties, to emphasize the dangers of carrying imaginative conviction in an age of uniform materialism. You hear about something happening in books or music through a friend, the aliveness of it, and certainly not through criticism. The latter pays homage to the reductionist views of the status quo, safety at all costs, the critic defining his limitations and not the vision under discussion. The ball is always on the other side of the wall. The critic can't see it, he never will. By failing to imagine, he reads himself and not the book.

Let us come back to the image, that fluent inner event which allows the poem to live, that happening in inner space which is the discourse of psyche. The image exists as an intermediary between inner and outer, it is an informing agent, one that alerts consciousness to archetypal or psychic components. When one freaks out, when the images implode autonomously across consciousness, we grow distressed at the speed and disorder of their arrival. It is like an agoraphobic person facing the West End crowds, someone drummed by panic in the city centre. The room opens to reveal a reservoir, a dead horse bleeds on the carpet, one's jet of urine prints out apocalyptic messages in its expiring arc. There is an accompanying panic at the fear of being alone and facing the future without someone there to right the spin. And out on the street it is worse. Do dark glasses help to hide disturbance? Who is the malevolent individual who fixes one with his eyes, as if he has been waiting for this moment of paranoid vulnerability in his victim for a long time? There is always a face in the crowd who would lay one out on the pavement.

My way of meeting the world is one of openness to all experience. Some drugs expand consciousness, attune perception to the suprareal, but most create their own pharmaceutical microcosm, a world of chemically generated responses rather than emotionally experienced impressions. Drugs leave one cut off – thirty thousand miles backstage in one's head. Inside that space one is fascinated by the unreal connections. The voltage flickers, current gets trapped, but it all takes place on the inside, with no other spectator than qualitative subjectivity. Being high often means self-gratification, self-communication, not extending boundaries beyond inner immediacy. The drug is the non-extensible trip. And so much is forgotten in the process, but so too are the experiences that filter through day consciousness.

Fear again tonight, that feeling of a black lake being sunk into my abdomen. There is no draining away this depth; I am the face staring up at an obsidian surface. On bad days I can't remember when the last line I wrote of this book ended and the next began. To sleep in the interval on the trail of words, but not sleep so much as stare wide-eyed at an off-white wall on which words write themselves in blood. And isn't madness a process of being unable to close the inner lens? It is a dysfunction of editing, seeing too much, and entering into a state of fixation with images that in another mind would be generated through dream. The red octopus emerging from cracks in the pavement, its tentacles swarming for the psychotic's wrist and jugular, stringing its suction pads to emaciated flesh, would be accepted within dream space as a valid if disturbing oneiric phenomenon. The intolerable image wakes the dreamer, there is a need to escape, crash out of the threatening dimension and retrieve familiar fixtures, the pillow, the ceiling, the bedside lamp, whatever we associate with daytime reality. But what about suspended dimension? Neither sleep nor waking, night nor day consciousness, an intermediary state in which the condition resembles trance or intoxication. The gravitation towards black-out after heavy drinking, or the period in which the drug hit decreases in intensity, has the user spaced into a blank, or the moment in which we think we might be asleep, but aren't, are signposts to the intermediary dimension. 'I saw nobody coming, so I went instead' as John Berryman has it in his sighting of absence, his filling in the space that the body becomes when we choose to be personalized.

Altered states of consciousness are directly linked to the creative principle. An art that defines reason does nothing to shift ways of seeing, it simply reports on a received universe. And what seems central to the individual's survival, whether the experience encountered is drug-induced or not, is directing the transforming energy rather than being manipulated by it. Most good art and writing siphon madness as a source, but the quantum balance between creator and pathology is one in which the artist stands outside the consuming circle. For the psychotic there is no distinguishing reality. For the poet there is a qualitative distinction between drawing on psychotic phenomena and the return to reality. This experience is also what we call shamanism and primitive magic. Stealing fire and living to tell the tale.

3

Withdrawal is synonymous with rebirth or regeneration of the neurology. Once the brain begins to produce its natural chemicals again, substances such as endorphins and the hormone adrenalin, the user acquires the confidence to be free of the habit. The processes of addiction and withdrawal are so subjectively interiorized in their subject that medicine makes a connection with this symbiosis only through the user's ability to articulate inner experience. The analyst wants to know my grammar of psychic awareness, the psychiatrist my biological tolerance to the substance. What I as the patient attempt to discover is how I shall differ when I am no longer dependent. I have known safety in my drugged parameters as well as paranoid threat. There has been insulation from reality, and a marked sense of dissociation has become a characteristic of my work. If drugs have a distinguishing mark, by which I mean that they set people apart as members of a particular chemical family, then that sense of difference is often what the user dreads relinquishing. The return to reality, a demystification in itself, is linked to a fear of anonymity. Are humans extraordinary? Most ideologies succeed in repressing individuation and subliminally implant the values to which its members are expected to subscribe. Drugs are one way of circumventing social dictates, creativity is another. Both are subversive acts in that they involve the re-creation of the universe. And therefore they return humans to the extraordinary, the underwater gardens in the unconscious where dolphins flip in and out of the open windows sunk in a coral château, and where the masked sleepwalker continues to juggle three orange cones as she drifts across the sands. And where is the authentic divide between inner and outer perception? Most of the time, even when we are engaged in close conversation with someone, we are somewhere else living with the incohesive stream of our inner dialogue.

No one's books better exemplify the direct link between dream and reality that André Breton's three experimental texts: *Nadja*, *L'amour fou* and *Arcane 17*. Deliberately unclassifiable as a genre, Breton's books shift effortlessly between fiction, reality, political reflection, discursive treatises on the transformative imagination, poetry and art. Breton's anti-novels take in everything pertinent to imaginative truth, and his analogical form lyricizes the extraordinary even where it is found in fact. Breton is arguably the greatest proponent of the imagination in that even his theory becomes imaginative thought. To the analogical mind that realizes the universe through the association of interconnected images, reality is an ideological monad that needs continually to be transcended by images as vital to life as planetary houses are to astrologers. 'For me,' says Breton, discussing the lives of subversively visionary poets 'the thing that was always passionately compelling about works like theirs was that they dropped a bombshell on their era, that they were created completely outside the cultural line of their ethos, and also that they pay much greater tribute than others to the aspirations and fears which form the common ground of humanity.'

It is on these volatile premises that the imagination builds. The outsider is the wolf in the high street. The poet dreaming of a new universe, the artist of the possibilities of form, and the junkie of a chemical nirvana, an alhambra located in the subway. Who hasn't walked through familiar streets of a city anticipating that at the next corner, down the alley where hookers are waiting under red lights, and to the left where a cinema has fallen into disuse, there will suddenly appear a turreted château with its lights reflected in the dark waters of a moat? Perhaps it is there owing to the union of chemicals, or the autonomous imploding of the imagination, or perhaps it has always been there, set apart by its forbidding walls, and only tonight presenting itself as a reality to the one who is attuned to its metaphor. Are there not two figures walking in the grounds? The woman is dressed in white and the man in red. They walk up stone steps towards a griffin partially obscured by ivy. They make love there and their turbulence twists like giant brushstrokes across the black water with the château's twenty illuminated rectilinear windows sunk in the lacquered surface.

NET, or neuro-electric therapy, the treatment devised by Dr Meg Patterson to counteract acute withdrawal symptoms, has proved to be one of the successful means of detoxification, and rock stars like Eric Clapton, Keith Richards and Pete Townshend have all benefited from its effects. Using a little black box which generates a tiny electrical current attuned to various frequencies, NET stimulates the production of the body's natural opiates. Drugs kill off the production of endorphins, and the black box allows the patient's regenerated defences the means to cope with withdrawal. NET helps the patient to level out over a period of four or five weeks, and is an effective means of obviating protracted withdrawal symptoms, and in the case of heroin addiction cold turkey. But users who elect to do it the slow way have to my mind not only a longer period in which to evaluate the transitional stages involved in a renascent neurology, a natural process in which to reflect on the neural library, but a surer means of encountering rebirth. Against this are the ferocity of panic attacks which so often make the patient revert to pharmaceuticals, and the whole vacillation over progress that this may entail. When one loses muscle tone, experiences fits of shaking, is doubled up unable to breathe, the temptation to have recourse to tablets that will correct panic symptoms is understandably acute.

My credit was little blue tablets, a benzodiazepine currency that trafficked with my chemistry. In the process of withdrawal I came to realize how the drug during addiction instates secondary symptoms that not only adopt the pattern of the original obsessions for which it was prescribed but intensify those symptoms so that the user regularly ups the quantity of the drug he is taking. The addict is feeding his need and not the anxiety that necessitated the drug being prescribed. And Ativan is bitter blue. The blues imply everything from Bessie Smith and Billie Holiday to solitary evenings waiting for a telephone call that never comes. Blue means watching a sultry *femme fatale* stand on the hotel terrace in a blue, sequinned dress, the hotel one is due to leave tomorrow; or it might mean autumn in the Black Forest; and it certainly suggests the down-mood slump that tranquillizers induce.

I should like to have met you, but I was right out of myself, dissociated. The summer lopes off like a dusty lion towards the equinox.

Taking drugs is the equivalent of missing time in terms of how UFO abductees report the experience. Years, months, days, whole blocks of time grow to be an unreality when your inner life is policed by chemicals. Monday is Wednesday or reverses back to Monday before being fast forwarded to Sunday. It is one way of breaking temporal chronology. It is one way of keeping clear of the pernicious routine involved in human life, for isn't employment the enemy of individuation and inner liberty? The system denies any alternative to linear time. UFO abductees speak of entering timelessness on contact, and of reverse electromagnetic fields killing time, and also of geographical transposition so that on release the abductee will sometimes find himself in a town hundreds of miles from his home. There is no accounting for this transition, there is only the gradual filling in of the amnesiac blank by the therapeutic help of hypnoregression. With drugs, that evaluative regression occurs during the period of withdrawal when the patient learns to reassemble the constituents of a former self. Who was I when I translated my emotions into chemical responses? I was not the person I am now, but my value of myself was different then. I believed like all addicts that my paranoid response to external events was the correct interpretation of reality despite the dramatic fluctuation of my moods. We can live only in the immediate, whatever impaired state of consciousness we bring to it. We need the objective admonition of someone close to us to help precipitate the move to get off drugs. We have to turn round in ourselves and see the damage, all the smoking car wrecks which are ditched off the side of the road.

In *Hooked?*, her book advocating the use of NET over all other methods of withdrawal, Meg Patterson documents the case of Susan, in her late thirties, who was assisted from her ten-year dependency on Ativan by treatment with NET. Her addiction was a circular trap, doctors encouraging her to continue with the drug rather than end up in casualty as a consequence of withdrawal. Learning to live without the drug demands a committed slice of one's life. GPs lack the time and psychological acumen to assist users to withdraw, and so it is up to the user to find a sympathetic support unit. Where do we go when we are ill? The question poses a conundrum. We all entertain the fantasy that there is someone somewhere in the world who has the knowledge and cure peculiar to our particular illness. This person will fulfil the subjective criteria necessary to being admitted to our private domain. But where do we find the elusive therapist? Indecisiveness is one of the many characteristics of addiction, so the initial search is unlikely to prove purposeful. There is every reason to delay. You can ask friends, you can go to local community centres to find numbers for helplines, but nothing is likely to approximate to the sensitive attention we have established as a fantasy need. Committing yourself for help to a stranger is a disquieting risk.

Wouldn't I like to find a cat-eyed Egyptian doctor, with mauve eyes and gold skin, who practises on the third floor of a white house overlooking the lake? She will treat her pharmacopoeia as an alchemical treatise. She will work by telemedical repair. Imbalance will be accessed and rectified. Her voice timbre will induce no trace of panic. The room will be dark green and the chairs dark blue. She has the knowledge to reprogram my billions of neural circuits. I can then choose to live and die at the flick of a karmic switch. 'I wish I could change my sex as I change my shirt,' wrote André Breton, and we all nurture the fantasy of needing to adopt a trial death for a while, but only on the condition that we can return if need be and switch over again in periods when life seems to be without potential for our particular desires.

Drugs more than anything are used to open up alternative realities and to present a parallel dimension to the user. If I say the poet should occupy a different reality each day, in that he is constantly remaking the universe through an imaginative alignment, and inhabiting that microcosm in preference to routine perception of things, this also holds good for those who use drugs to subvert the ideological manipulation of time. It is not idealism to presuppose that our little time should be used constructively and creatively rather than be channelled into deleterious systems of employment. But there is also an out of it, largely from heroin, which is a negative state of missing time. Guitarists like Keith Richards of the Rolling Stones, whose reckless abuse of drugs led to chronic heroin addiction, report blocks of life that were erased by a comatose response to every aspect of living. David Bowie speaks of having holes in his brain from his excessive use of cocaine in the early seventies, and of being unable to remember anything of the year he spent in Los Angeles in 1975. A year as a white blank: the big sleep. His psychophysical health entered a period of alarming dissolution: he lined cocaine on a mirror with a hundred-dollar bill, lived in a dark room with pentagrams splashed on the walls as symbols of occult protection, and even went so far as to store his urine in the refrigerator, a precaution Aleister Crowley took against being magically subverted. Acute paranoia combined with fluctuating periods of hyperactivity and its counterpart depression, and the delusion that his mind was being worked upon by an underground occult group, brought Bowie to the edge of disintegration. There is even an authenticated report that the house in which Bowie was staying, called The House on Doheney, was the subject of an isolated rainstorm, the rest of the street remaining in clear and uninterrupted white sunlight.

Bowie imagined also at the time that if a woman were to get pregnant from him she would give birth to the Antichrist. He came to believe that he was a walk-in, an alien whose sensitivities were too brutally exposed to a manipulative public. And those whose gifts contribute to altering world consciousness need advanced psychic protection: a gravitation to drugs and alcohol is seen as part of a necessary defence. If you are a reluctant incarnation rather than a humanoid, and a palpably sensitive interpreter of consciousness rather than an alien, life can appear too overtly hostile. And drugs or alcohol just happen. There may be no preconceived ritual attached to their taking; it is more probable that at some stage they occurred and became an inextricable part of that person's life. If it was pressure that triggered Bowie's habit, very soon it became inseparable from his neurology. What happens in private in a performer's life are the facts that are concealed from the public by way of their translation into direct biography. It is the scenes, the intractable paranoia, the scheming duplicities committed for money, the illnesses, the propping up of someone totally dependent that are the daily routine. Bowie was not only feeding a cocaine habit but was drinking ferocious quantities of vodka. He was hospitalized twice in Berlin in 1976 for alcoholism and suspected suicide attempts.

It took Bowie until the eighties to get clear and to adjust to a way of life not contingent on toxins. Having established a cult of being in touch with aliens right from the release of 'Space Oddity' early on in his career, and maintaining that persona through his clothes and androgyny (his eyes are two distinctly different colours, and one is marginally out of alignment), Bowie appeared to be the progenitor of a humanoid species. A role which, owing to the delusional character transformations brought about by cocaine, he was not unwilling to adopt. His brain underwent a chemical apocalypse. He incorporated futuristic cityscapes into his stage sets and played the role of an alien in Nicolas Roeg's film *The Man Who Fell to Earth*, his imaginal fantasies taking on a schizoid embodiment in which he saw himself personified as the cocaine-dazed rock star. By 1975 he had grown to be so emaciated that death looked imminent. A Giacometti sculpture in white make-up, Bowie's profile was that of a chemicalized androgyne. And there are those who would argue that his finest work was inspired by drugs and that the avant-garde experiments he released on 'Low' in 1977 advanced his pharmaceutical-inspired theories to an exhaustive conclusion. The trajectory expired on a curve in imaginative space. The post-drugs Bowie symbolized by his commercial ventures in the eighties seemed singularly lacking in the innovative creative energies with which he had dynamized an earlier decade.

Coming off drugs involves a complex metamorphosis. For Bowie it entailed a certain demystification of appearance and a readiness to compete with commercial strains of music rather than live out on an angular edge. Drugs are a solo experience, and because of that singularity of isolation which they generate artists sometimes appear freer to experiment with inner conviction rather than modify that vision for collective approval. But there is a balance needed here: too much insularity and the effects achieved may prove solipsistic; what is required is the right combination of inner and outer realities. Artaud tried everything: opium, hashish, peyote and heroin. He navigated a paranoid channel through a black sea, but his tone is always exalted and direct, no matter its hostility to all forms of bourgeois convention. It declares with passionately lyric rage that we seek vision as an ultimate value. In his short essay 'Opium et sécurité générale' Artaud argues in favour of the mad, the visionary and the degenerate as being a privileged order set apart from humanity. 'Unfortunately for illness, medicine does exist,' he tells us, before arguing that drugs should be made available to the few because the majority would gain little from their use. 'And you, lucid madmen, consumptives, cancer-ridden, chronic meningitics, you are the misunderstood. There is a point in you that no doctor will ever understand and it is the point which, for me, saves you and makes you majestic, pure and marvellous: you are outside life, you are above life, you have pains which the ordinary man does not know, you go beyond the normal level and that is why men are against you, you are poisoning their quiet, you are the dissolvers of their stability.'

Artaud's inspirited credo, aligning drugs with the visionary impulse, was of course taken up by Burroughs and the Beat generation. Drugs were seen as a countermeasure to repressive societal conventions. Man's great liberty lies in the inexhaustible reserves of inner space. How you connect with your own cellular chemistry determines where you travel in terms of expanding areas of consciousness. The alchemists in their allegorical sensitization of inner states worked towards the achievement of ascendant gold. Psychic potential in human beings is realized through the channelling of creative energies and by tapping into an image-pool which is the metaphoric equivalent of oneiric gold. I write a poem and I retrieve a codification of images which were previously unprocessed in my psyche. Creativity when it is imaginatively directed is like a continuous march on the hidden gold mines at the interior. We go in search of excavating the great inner secrets. The addict arrives there by different ways, and is sometimes too disorientated to master the latent material he is in the process of discovering.

When I was withdrawing I felt hunted by a figure who came to adopt and represent a composite identity. The person was a man with high shoulders, coarsely aggressive features and dressed in a black greatcoat. He had been wounded and dripped a spotted trail of blood from a source hidden by his greatcoat. Although he walked directly towards me, never narrowing or increasing the distance he had chosen to set us apart, it was the nature of the hunt that he never caught up with me. But manifested in his person was explosively repressed aggression, and a knowledge on my part that he had found me out. He knew my secret. Whatever deep inner terror I had sunk in the bottom of a lake, he had found. I would see his blood-spots on the pavement, a long snake-tailed thread receding to the Hampstead woods. At night I was afraid he would break down my windows and doors, or I would draw back a curtain to find him looking in at me. Eluding a reality that is invisible to others leads to acute paranoia. One lives with the fear that others will confirm the reality of what is happening, and the additional disquiet that one may be trapped in a subjective prism. Where do I go from here? Munch's painting has something of an answer.

The case of the German writer Unica Zürn, the companion and lover of the surrealist artist Hans Bellmer, and who in 1970 threw herself from the sixth-floor window of their apartment in Paris, presents one of the richest studies of a private fantasy world in contention with reality. Like Anna Kavan, Unica Zürn created a personal world of archetypal associations, and one in which metamorphoses of persons and things became the shape-changing vocabulary of her inner discourse. Zürn went in and out of mental clinics and lived in anticipation of creative 'miracles', as she called them. She detached herself by invariably writing in the third person, her world being one in which reality has no recognizable frontiers. Things change shape, any accidental encounter may trigger off a series of synchronistic associations, and a hostility to psychiatric medicine is voiced with an acrimonious disgust which sometimes recalls Artaud's obsessive rage at the electroshock therapy administered to him at Rodez.

In her *L'homme-jasmin* Zürn encounters her childhood fantasy figure, the mescaline proponent and writer Henri Michaux, as a reality, and having personalized her fiction and found what she assumed to be the ideal husband, she dips out of control into a world of unmodified hallucination. Zürn writes the poetic commentary on her split, and dissolves all barriers between inner and outer realities. Even gender becomes transformed by her particular way of seeing.

> Both have been afflicted by an incredible transformation. Under the observation of the psychiatrists and nurses, and with the help of injections, the man will turn slowly into a woman and the woman into a man. They will feel themselves saved, and marry. As she leaves her bedroom she sees her friend who has gone out on to the veranda. He doesn't even look at the sky. He doesn't see the enormous crocodile. He doesn't see images of the past rolling by in the clouds. He doesn't see the pure forms of the baroque era, despite his passion for that genre. He doesn't number amongst the initiates and the elect.

Zürn's writings are pure examples of autonomous hallucination. Things are experienced rather than described. The action of her work is dependent on the condition of her illness. There are writers who set out to establish madness by descriptive states, and there are those whose work is that encounter. Zürn's work follows in the tradition of Nerval's *Aurélia*, Lautréamont's *Maldoror*, Breton's *Nadja*, Desnos's *Liberté ou l'amour*, Leonora Carrington's *Down Below* and Dali's *Hidden Faces* in that all these works subvert by a form of archetypal insurrection and demand that we accept their implosive interiors as a legitimate and equally authentic expression of reality. No apology is asked for underworld culture. And is not Sade in his fantastic cataloguing of sexual atrocities, most of them imagined as happening behind the sealed walls of castles, one of the original creators of the hallucinated novel? The Divine Marquis tilted a welcome shadow across the future of a novel written to confirm the premises of social realism.

Zürn's analogical method of writing creates a displacement in which counter-reality assumes dominance. Her prose is concentrated, as of someone watching a film inside her head. Reality is not necessary, it is on the other side of viewing. What she sees are numerals, anagrammatic puzzles, midgets the size of her thumb, eagles, deformation in faces, and an explosively apocalyptic epilogue to even the simplest practical functions. If psychiatrists could implant a video camera in the stream of psychotic phenomena generated by someone with a creative focus like Unica Zürn, something of the nature of inner reality would confirm the authenticity of the visionary.

Zürn's imagination is filmic, and her visuals follow on one from the other with brilliant clarity:

> A red lacquer scorpion fell from the air and landed on the plate with an evil, clattering noise. Without stopping to deliberate on the matter, I crushed it underneath a small stone Buddha statue I found beside the plate. The splintering rage with which it expired was replaced by a glassy shriek as I threw it into the fire. White wings fluttered through the open window. A white eagle bowed before me, and for a moment I felt myself being embraced in its pinions. Its magnificent blue eyes just looked at me with pride and audacity.

These implosively kinetic happenings are a reality and occur with a sequential clarity which suggests that imaginal mythemes are part of a highly processed narrative. Psychiatry imposes a language on creative discovery which seems to have little in common with the fluent association that writers like Unica Zürn establish through the hallucinated imagination. The problem is always one of trying to situate consciousness. Who and where are we in relation to inner and outer activity? If we align predominantly through inner activity and accord dominance to that function, we are often considered disturbed or mad. If we elect to live and place our locus in the interior, we are considered to be violating social taboo. We are not entering into discourse with a shared reality. The drug user similarly offends, for taking drugs is seen as an antisocial dictate, and one that bypasses participation in the material world. And it is a matter of psychological predisposition as to which we find the most interesting. If we are inner, we grow secret and preoccupied with what is happening on the inside. Parents and disciplinarian adults can't get at our amazingly fertile elaboration of the inner story.

Even without a heightened awareness of free associated imagery we are dual creatures. We switch over at night from waking consciousness to unconsciousness and the dream journey. The creative are those who can accede to the oneiric source without being in dream states. Surrealism, or psychic automatism as Breton defines it, is simply dreaming with your eyes open. For Breton dreams and reality are a direct connecting current, whereas for Freud the two are in a relation of conflicting displacement. The receptive trance state that Breton advocates is not so very different, Octavio Paz points out, from the pure condition of Buddhist meditation in which images are allowed to be generated autonomously from the unconscious. Breton's needs though were not those of the passive contemplative; they belonged to those of the dynamized sensibility that imposes poetic order on the chaotic and presents the material as a disturbing alternative to reasoned control. If I see a big red fish sail over in the clouds, or a girl in the street change to a green-eyed, leopard-spotted creature belonging to the world of metamorphic archetypes, if I see my hand turn gold and a number of people gathered on a ledge in the sky, that is the reality which is dominant. It is my vision, and in the process of seeing I displace the familiar world around me.

Unica Zürn's transmogrifying vision has her constantly switching channels in terms of reality. Fictionalizing one of her stays in St Anne's Hospital, Zürn, like all patients suffering from projective hallucination, wonders whether it is the drugs given to her or her state of mind that contributes to the confusion in which she finds herself.

> Once she has had her first *interrogatoire* with the young psychiatrist, the staff decide which sedatives she is to be prescribed: Haloperidol, Keithon and Nozinan; these medications cause her to hallucinate, or is that dependent on her morbid

state? When she lies on her bed, she fixes her eyes on the wardrobe's fibreglass doors and sees a constant relay of faces, animals and landscapes which keep changing expression as part of a continuous film. These hallucinations, which are similar to her interpretations of the patterns in the doors, frighten her just as much as they fascinate. Gradually it grows to be obsessive, and whenever she goes into the garden to escape the wardrobe doors and sit on a bench in the sun, she begins to see fantastic creatures moving through the grass and the simple meadow flowers. She cannot stand this state any longer and asks the doctor to up her doses of Nozinan, a drug she has grown accustomed to over the years.

We are faced here with the familiar agonized dilemma of the patient who can bear neither reality. What you are seeing on the inside is insufferable, and the outer is no more tolerable. Very often one repeats the other, and the hallucinated duality of seeing generates hysteria. Then there is nowhere to go. Closing or opening the eyes give on to the same hallucinated terror. It is then that the skin bristles as though a wolf has found its way into the room at night, despite the locked doors, the barred windows. A wolf carrying a red bone in its teeth which it deposits at your feet.

Unica Zürn's courage, as it has been with so many creative artists, was to observe her own disintegration and to write down those experiences as a narrative of polymorphous breakdown. Pathological diagnoses result in a biologized formula for madness, whereas the creative impulse goes beyond those strictures and works with the condition as a process of transformation. When Zürn eventually committed suicide it was as a means of opposing one mania with another – the hysterical force of her trajectory from the window of her Paris apartment was her only means of extinguishing the dual inner and outer paranoiac visions that had pursued her throughout her life. And it was Henri Michaux, a writer largely influenced by hallucinogens, who was her obsession, a poet I shall have reason to look at later on in this study.

How we release or somatize the pain that could potentially

lead to a habit depends on the individual sensibility and how we direct our energies. The iconic image of self-destructive degradation associated with rock stars often leads to the idolization of junkies. Keith Richards of the Rolling Stones is a pertinent example. His addiction to smack throughout the seventies resulted in his being arrested in Canada in the course of a 1977 tour. Prior to his arrest he had gone to Switzerland to have blood transfusions so that no trace of the drug could be discerned by toxicologists monitoring his entry into America. When he was apprehended for the massive quantities of heroin discovered in his hotel bedroom, his only means of avoiding incarceration was voluntarily to undergo withdrawal and to donate a million dollars to drug-related charities.

What is important here is how a drug was mythologized by the user going public. Pharmaceuticals are consumed and metabolized, and if we guess by the notation of someone's physical reactions that they are on drugs, still the issue remains private. Forced by the authorities to undergo a cure, Richards's management contacted Dr Meg Patterson about the potentially painless methods of disengagement that NET offered. In Richards's own words: 'It's so simple. It's a little metal box with leads that clip on to your ears and in two or three days – which is the worst period for kicking junk – in these seventy-two hours it leaves your system.' Chronic withdrawal syndrome is obviated by the use of a particular frequency for a particular drug. This rapid method of detoxification, the electricity serving to cleanse the system and assist the brain in processing its own chemicals, is a means back to reality, the starting-point from which the patient must then reconstruct a purposeful life. Dysphoria is the natural accompaniment to withdrawal, a sense of craving and psychological maladjustment making the subject feel at a tilt to the world. One projects one's own shadow and sits in that penumbra.

Richards seems to have kicked heroin after having been successfully treated by NET, but then to have substituted liquor for drugs, his legendary consumption of Jack Daniel's displacing one toxic excess with another. And this is a pattern pursued by most junkies, the majority graduating to whisky as a stimulus to and alleviant from cellular craving.

Two days ago I started seeing fire again. It was up in the tree-tops as a reddish swirl catching yellow. I could hear the whiplash of its consuming crackle. A visual and audio-hallucination or a reality? What I had on the phenomenon though was a slight distance. I was not going to be directly burnt. The thing had reappeared because I was undergoing a period of nervous exhaustion, a dislocation from fluent energy. My spatial relationship to the fire was one of warning. I was being told to slow the period of overreach, the manic rush that so often accompanies the writing of a book. When I am writing I am over-conscious of the translation of inner material into time. I have the construct of the book inside and the work required to liberate it into language is a temporal thing. This is the inexorably redoubtable aspect of writing. I know it but I have to say it, inner to outer, and the quantum leap involves work with its corresponding exaggeration of time. I am already sighting the last word, but I am still on p. 69.

Henri Michaux, poet, traveller, artist and pioneer of mescalin experimentation, was as mentioned earlier the fixed obsession of Unica Zürn. Imagining him first, and living with him as a psychotic fiction of her own invention, she was later to encounter him as a reality in Paris and to form an intense liaison with him. Michaux's writings and accompanying anxiety drawings are an attempt to notate interiority as it is perceived through hallucinogens. Michaux's advance is on the illusorily infinite; he dynamizes the visionary impulse to cut every way to the interior. He attempts to reorganize our way of sighting inner and outer realities. Michaux is the would-be progenitor of a new neurophysiological species. His deconstruction of finite limitations demands new physical premises: android, humanoid, alien connotations. He is compelled by an inner gravity field to march on another sun, another system of planets. He is a deep space voyager whose returns to reality find him disorientated by familiar signs and repetitions. He experimented with innumerable drugs, each affording a different reality, and gave expression to his findings through his multi-art forms.

Michaux has placed an exact faith in hallucination. In his book *L'infini turbulent* he emphasizes the greater reality of hallucination and its reliability in transmitting truth. 'Hallucinations', he writes, 'are infinitely more real than the sight of ordinary reality. Reality, being formed of contradictory elements and impressions, is open to doubt, distracting, fragmentary. It diverts one's attention. It is seen to be there largely as an obstacle. As for hallucinations, they are resonantly synergic, synthetic, global, and in their perfect and concentrated, exact correspondence with the idea, the aspiration, the fear, the inner image, they are indisputable. THEY FIT.'

Michaux's described notion that reality is there as an obstacle to truth is of course the shared conviction of visionary poets. Baudelaire had begun it all with his declared ennui from two-dimensional living and his pathological disillusionment with reality. The attempt thereafter amongst a few solitary disaffected individuals was to use poetry as a means of discovering new worlds. Lautréamont and Rimbaud both furnished this aim, an intention concentrated and intensified by the surrealists, and Michaux as an antecedent to the Beats took up a maverick itinerary in the hallucinated universes of drug exploration.

Without ever being affiliated to surrealism, Michaux shares with Breton and his associates the notion of subverting ideological reality by the discovery of imaginal worlds. Interiors created by psychic autonomy are retrieved from the unconscious. Michaux's world is one in which anything and everything may happen. Images are the currency of hallucination, and good poetry sets up an electromagnetic field of associations between image valencies. Michaux's spiral embraces the primal, the apocalyptic and the futuristic. Octavio Paz tells us: 'Michaux does not invent: he sees. He astonishes us because he shows us what is hidden in the creases of our souls. All those creatures inhabit us, live and sleep with us. We are at the same time the fields they cultivate and their battlefields.'

One senses that Michaux, in the manner of William Burroughs and Brion Gysin, used his physical body as a lab for experiments. No matter the nausea or discomfort induced by a drug, Michaux continues to observe its effects, and the inner spaces it opens up to vision. There is a clinical detachment from his organism which is there also in Burroughs, the presupposition being one of the body's apparent indestructibility. States are encountered in the interests of vision. Users of hallucinogens are the great cosmonauts; they go to reclaim undiscovered interiors in the way that adventurers sailed into the blue in search of the world's finite boundaries. Readers of Terence McKenna's *True Hallucinations* will encounter experiences demanding a temerity and visionary courage belonging to no other order than those who risk life and sanity to pursue Michaux's concept of infinity or plural worlds.

So connected are the correlations of inner and outer space, that Michaux speaks of encountering black images or black visions, the equivalent of black holes in space: 'Suddenly I am frightened. I have just seen black images. And what if blackness were to extend for ever? What if, outside myself as within myself, I were to find that I was immersed in black? I am invaded by blobs, covering me in their multiplicity, and clouding over my sky. The habitual cleft rocks are black, so are the monuments that vibrate without falling, and heads are black like obsidian. And so it begins, until a seething inhabits space.'

Michaux relates the states of hysteria, delirium, dystopia and ecstasy which overtake him in the course of tripping on mescalin. He engages psychophysically with the drug and its corresponding levels of expansion and contraction. He opens himself to every form of chemical permutation and writes and draws direct out of the immediate experience. His inner explorations are heroic. He is constantly opening doors into inner space. He somatizes the word and transmits it into his angular, nervous line. He gets into his work only what is vital to the imagination. All lesser substance is eliminated. Michaux's work is remarkable for its clear focus. He places absolute faith in his retrieval of inner states. He sees himself as a cosmic voyager and sometimes as an explorer navigating the still uncharted seas of the imagination. In *Misérable miracle* he writes of encounters with aquatic imagery:

> At times thousands of little ambulacral tentacles of a gigantic starfish fastened to me so completely that I could not tell if I was becoming the starfish or if the starfish had become me. I contracted, I made myself watertight, but compression opens

out to relaxation again, even the enemy dissolves like salt in water, and once more I was predominantly navigation, shining with a pure white flame, responding to a thousand cascades, to foaming rifts and to gyratory gougings. . . . The streaming torrents that poured through me on this remarkable day were so unforgettably unique that I thought – (I never stopped thinking) 'A mountain, in spite of its unintelligence, a mountain with its cascades, its ravines, its bubbling slopes would be in the same state as I am in now, and better able to understand me than a man. . . .'

The contention between inner and realist literature has existed for centuries, and it is a profoundly staged conflict. In large a rationalistic social literature predominates as the populist genre. It has the support of critical opinion which is there to maintain the status quo, but its measures are short-lived and confined to the media system promoting it. It is the inner voice, usually condemned to go underground, that is responsible for the individual risk, making an art that outlives itself. Rimbaud's solitary and at the time suppressed voice has succeeded in extinguishing successive generations of sociably acceptable poets. Blake waged war on his contemporaries from mythological space, Hart Crane ran up against the punitively restrictive critical myopia of his age, but a generation of French writers which included Michaux were successful from Dada onwards in bending the creative axis inwards, and in presenting inner space as the richest medium of creative expression. In other words it is the true reality, or dreaming with your eyes open. Michaux is in every sense of the word a cartographer. Today we draw up moon maps, Mars maps, Jupiter maps, blueprints of the nearer planets. Michaux monitors a parallel universe he explored in his unconscious. He was always getting there, he was always arriving, not only for the time the drug stayed in his body, but for a whole life of poetic reflection on implosive phenomena. His initial texts were written and drawn chaotically under the influence of hallucinogens, and in reflection he would add an imaginative coherency to a primal text. His work vibrates with wave-image and wave-thought frequencies. He voluntarily enters into states that bear parallels with schizophrenic and psychotic phenomena. He hallucinates the object of a foetus sitting in the wash-basin. His panic is terrible. It is a membranous red and blue. The power of the seer uniting with the seen makes him constantly anxious to differentiate between hallucination and reality. He wants to experience the indivisibility of the two perceptions, but at the same time he has to make the distinction in order to evaluate that difference in his writing. The tension in his work comes about from his describing discoveries made on the inside. Michaux needs dualities, he celebrates the transformative powers of the drug and of the imagination and in doing so establishes a new universe. He sees a glass ladder telescoping to the stars, he is terrified by the compact thunder of wings beating in his head, his tongue grows into a pink hippopotamus, colour implodes across his vision, he is invaded by unrecognizable faces. He is the man who finds himself sitting on the inside of a world he can never reach. He can enter into the fluency of his vision but he can never properly retain it except through words or line interpretation. And they are the cooling afterthought to the wave-line of his hallucinated imagery. Michaux seeks speed through mescalin. He drives poetry like a Lamborghini. He zips through the fluctuating phases of imagery the drug generates, while all the time being conscious that his mind is being fuelled by the limitations of his body.

Autohypnotized by his visions, Michaux was aware of touching on the peripheries of madness, and often of walking round a circle of fire: 'Now I understand. In this moment of distress it reminds me of madness and is itself the very image of madness: a lit circle and everything else in shadow. This is it: the alluring circle from which escape is impossible and where something appears to you alone, cutting you off from the rest. This is what it is, a rope tightening around the neck, obvious to everyone except you.'

The terror associated with madness and drug experience, and by extension the creative state, is the lack of preconceived correlates available to the mind. Nothing has prepared you for the big terror. It seems inconceivable that faces in the street may appear bloody, lacerated, pulped like a scooped water-melon. And how is it that there is a noise in the sky that only you can hear? Why does a particular tone of red or yellow make you feel instantly nauseated? And that side-street. You know if you go down it you will meet with murder. There's a blood-stained shirt in the gutter, a rat poking around a mashed carton, a smell of leather in the oppressive air. Everything vibrates with potential menace when you are strung out on attenuated nerves. Parallel dimensions open up, into which you may disappear. Why are there suddenly shop mannequins standing amongst the trees? They weren't there before. And that Boeing has its port wing on fire as it descends into the glideways. These are weird days you never expected to know. There's a grave dug in the middle of the road. You know that person's face, and there's a car approaching.

Michaux saw drug taking as an 'infinity mechanism', a process that extracted him from time, in the way that Cocteau took opium in order to get off the speeding train and sit on the bank. If we are preoccupied in life with a calling that seems rapidly to consume our days without allowing time for reflection, we search for some means of slowing down the rush. Drugs may seem to present a more dynamized form of inner expression than meditation or the various forms of yoga, but that quality is subjective and contingent on a person's psychic potential. There are no short cuts to creative vision, but there are drugs that will facilitate means to self-illumination and provide pointers to the hidden geography of the unconscious.

Michaux was so attuned to his neurological library that he wrote and drew simultaneously with the drug's own rhythm in his biochemistry. 'The quick vibrating lines I drew endlessly, without thinking, without hesitating, without pausing, by their very appearance tended towards a "visionary" drawing.' But in the process of his experiments Michaux risked madness. He tells us in *Misérable miracle* that on one occasion he miscalculated the quantity of mescalin he was using and faced dementia as a consequence. He suddenly felt responsible for keeping a close watch on the psychopath who had come to occupy his mind. He felt threatened by the alien who had come to inhabit his consciousness. In flipping he had produced his shadow side. He had become someone else, a brutal walk-in, an intraperson, an intruder in his own psychophysical space.

> The lamp by the mirror showed me a face I had never seen before, that of a raving madman. It would have frightened a murderer. It would have had him run away. Frantic, brutally extroverted, coolly photogenic and resolved on its purpose, it was the face of someone possessed, though neither the face nor I had moved. It was the mask of a person who no longer listens, a psychopath's face, a man, that is, mad with fear. The vicious face was that of a wild animal's at bay.

Michaux's encounter with the other belongs to the category of displacement obsessions that threaten the phobic and those undergoing hallucinatory terror. We are without warning inhabited by an opposite or some tangential entity that has shown up on the inside. In a state of pathological breakdown I dreaded becoming a depotentiated rebirth, a simulacrum of all I most feared. I would imagine my hands and feet as twice their size, my body square, and my face developing the features of a lycanthropic wolf-man. I would never be myself again, according to the psychological fantasy.

Where do we go and what do we do when we encounter obsessive states? Michaux writes in *Misérable miracle* of how for several weeks, owing to a reverse reflex, he had to avoid taking a familiar walk by the Seine for fear he would push someone into the river. He would live out the reality as a fantasy, a shadow murder that took place in his head, but without the clear distinction we usually make between events that happen on the inside and impulses which are externalized into actions. The obsessive may keep on rerouting his car in the attempt to retrieve the body he is sure he has hit, or in advanced schizoid states phobic guilt may exist that the person has committed psychopathic crimes, and no amount of external evidence to the contrary will act as a countermeasure.

Drugs, creativity, obsessive phobic conditions, hallucination, all of these expressions belong in some way to modified or unmodified psychotic phenomena. Where is the distinction between imagination and pathology? I would argue that artists are those who channel the psychic components of breakdown into articulate form. The occupation involves risk. When the volume gets turned up too high, there is a possibility of audiovisual overload. And madness is a process of seeing what the artist anticipates. Dali's and Ernst's landscapes, and the interiors of most surreal paintings whether they are by Magritte, Yves Tanguy or Giorgio de Chirico, juxtapose images that belong pathologically to the world of paranoid schizophrenia. What the creative sensibility gives to the world of psychiatry and psychology is the presentation of images retrieved from incipient pathology, isolating them for analytical scrutiny. The artist often creates a parallel universe that approximates to the idea of madness. The junkie asserts less control over the experience, and is in part a passive spectator to involuntary chemical associations. The paranoid schizophrene or the psychotic are the victims of unchannelled phenomena which are also translated into physical dysfunctions. The visionary poet from Rimbaud right through the twentieth century has subscribed to a 'systematic derangement of the senses', a voluntary pact with altered states of consciousness generated by what Breton called psychic automatism. When I write, I denormalize; I open myself to the potential for madness which lives in me. The notion of inspired poetry, whether it is conceived of as shamanic or daimonic possession, demands a sense of autonomous journey. Writing that keeps to rational consciousness fails to excite, for the absence of transformative energies suggests the writer's inability to connect with chaos. And the process is a psychophysical one involving the body as vehicular springboard to creative expression. The poet uses hysteria, but without the spontaneous body language that invests the clinical hysteric. Hillman is excellent on the subject: 'Hysteria somatizes consciousness. A classical conversion hysteria converts psychic meanings into somatic demonstrations: the central idea is acted, the intelligible account of things converts back into the ritual dromenon; psychic events become body events; meanings enter behaviour. . . . Hysterical reactions may be seen as desperate attempts to refind body, to incarnate, to find initiation into life.'

Initiation into life is most often through breakdown. Madness is like visiting a hooker. You go in and you come out changed. There is a new way of seeing and interpreting experience. Imagine the red light, and follow.

4

'Heartbreak Hotel', the blue atmospheric lyric that Elvis Presley made famous as a song, contains the line 'Down the end of Lonely Street'. Lonely Street is where the mad as well as the broken-hearted go. You never expect to visit the place, make no preparations for the event, take no suitcases, you just find yourself there and later on piece together the fragments of the mosaic leading to your arrival. It is usually raining. A blue rain. Sometimes the people have faces without features. Dogs pick through garbage in the streets. Soggy books, rubies and old photographs litter the pavements. The street is an impasse. You can't find any sense of identity. Your papers have disappeared. The pill bottles in your pockets are empty. The hooker outside the hotel has her hair gelled like Presley's and carries a red cardboard heart. The taxi that crawls down the street has no driver behind the wheel. There is a craving in you that is like cellular explosion. Amnesic patches alternate with manic implosion. You are too tired ever to sleep again. There is only one place to go: the blue, neon-lit hotel. But when you arrive in the entrance hall the desk-clerk is slumped over with a bullet-hole through his right temple. The stairs have been demolished. Spiders run in zigzag spirals across the fissured floor. There is a discarded blue suede shoe in the foyer. The rat that comes out of the cupboard walks on its hind legs and is taller than you. It has purple eyes. You realize you haven't been breathing for so long you could be swimming underwater. It doesn't seem to matter anyway. It is too late to revise the mechanism. Maybe you are dead and clearing through hallucinatory states before the light shines through. That doesn't matter either. You have visited Heartbreak Hotel. The hooker is still smiling at you.

There is in Anna Kavan's fiction an extraordinary sense of displaced identity, a sort of multi-channelled consciousness that switches from one reality to another without ever being sure of an exact location. Kavan's figures, like Kafka's, enter a labyrinthine mirror world in which familiar signs are metamorphosed into alien concepts. Nothing in Kavan's world is fixed. Her way of seeing is shape-lifting and hallucinatory. It is in Kavan's post-war fiction that her inimitable, partly drug-induced vision of a frontierless world anticipates the concerns of sci-fi futurists like J.G. Ballard and William Burroughs. Kavan was addicted to heroin as early as 1926, long before the substance grew to be a fashionable street drug, and her addiction continued until the time of her death in 1968. For most of that time she was dependent on private prescriptions from Dr Karl Bluth, who continued to legitimize the drug for her use until his death in 1964. Kavan was largely unaware that a whole drug cult had developed around smack with the publication of Burroughs's *Naked Lunch*, and the media promotion of the youth culture centred upon rock music. Highly individual, deeply private, and one of the true originals of mid-century British writing, Kavan inhabited a personalized and fantastic universe. She is not only a marvellous antidote to a fiction of social realism, but a courageous inner explorer who encountered madness as a consequence of her fertile imagination. Kavan has the outsider's inveterate disrespect for literary fashions. She is never anything but herself, and like all writing that travels to the interior her later poetic prose dispenses with formulated props like character development and thematic conclusions. Her books are like life, unreal and open-ended. They move effortlessly between dream and reality.

Kavan is obsessed with unpredictable intersections. The stranger who comes out of nowhere, the double, the figure concealed by the ordinary landscape are all metaphors for madness. Things are not as they seem, they never are. 'A neatly dressed man with a bag in his hand is hurrying along the street to the station. His arrival is timed very well as the smoke of the train can be seen in the distance just as he gets to the booking office. But then, instead of buying a ticket, he suddenly walks out of the station again, takes a piece of chalk out of his pocket, marks something on the door of one of the neighbouring houses, and hurries off in quite another direction.' This filmic incident from *Sleep Has His House* typifies Kavan's ability to create parallel universes. She transforms visual perception into narrative permutation. The eye systematically records, but seeing as it is known through the imagination goes beyond that register and creates the possibilities presented by the encounter. Good writing is about those possibilities, and what happens on the shadow side of experience. Kavan is rapacious for visual detail, her eye finds the visible and concealed particulars in any given scene. Her descriptive writing has the sensitivity of the best lyric poetry, and in almost all ways she is closer to the French writers of the *nouveau roman* than she is to her British contemporaries. Her concerns are with submerged threat, and her landscapes telescope from the seemingly innocuous domestic to the elementally apocalyptic. She arrives at places by fluent teleportation, and ice, which was to form the anonymous amnesiac landscape of one of her major novels, had much to do as an environmental image with the white powder she fed into her veins. Her prose is integrated, vibrant and plethoric with imagery. She is in the great line of inner explorers, and ends up in places that re-create the universe. She would have arrived at the same imaginative destinations without drugs, the unconscious material was always there, coded into her impulses. Heroin simply encouraged her to withdraw from life and deepen the time available to her creative resources. She found in the drug a conspiratorial angularity to life.

Kavan was registered with the Home Office as an addict, and over the years attempted detoxification in psychiatric units, but never successfully. Her biographer David Callard tells us of the implicit sexual aspect of her dependency on her psychiatrist Dr Bluth. 'The closest they came to sex, of a highly sublimated Freudian manner, was when Bluth administered her injections for her. He was the first doctor to realize the incurability of her addiction and the fact that heroin served as an antidote to her black, suicidal depressions. According to Raymond Marriott, [the theatre critic who became her friend and literary executor], all future detoxifications were undertaken, not with the goal of abstinence but to regulate a habit which had, for one reason or another, got out of control.'

Kavan destroyed all her private papers and journals, and the latter would doubtless have provided a deeply subjective record of her habit. But the novels afford us a metaphoric geography of her hallucinated imagination. Like that of J.G. Ballard, Kavan's vision takes in global transformation and the apocalyptic deterioration of our planet. The shifts are subtle and occur on an imaginative dimension which in time becomes representational reality. At the end of *Ice*, the glacial world encroaching on the recognized universe, there is an intensely moving passage in which the protagonist finds herself confined to the warm interior of a car, her last outpost against whiteness. The ice-wall is thought to be advancing as far as the equator, and the getaway from blizzarding cold is also seen as a hope for the imagination, a small human light travelling into the unknown.

> Driving the big car through the glacial night I was almost happy. I did not regret that other world I had longed for and lost. My world was now ending in snow and ice, there was nothing else left. Human life was over, the astronauts underground, buried by tons of ice, the scientists wiped out by their own disaster. I felt exhilarated because we two were alive, racing through the blizzard together. . . . The world seemed to have come to an end already. It did not matter. The car had become our world; a small, bright, heated room; our home in the vast, indifferent, freezing universe.

Writers such as Kavan drive the imagination like a car. The objective is to overtake oneself, and in doing so pursue a trajectory that jumps into a parallel dimension. In the last years of her life her work was enthusiastically taken up by a youth culture alert to drugs, rock music, space travel and an explorative concern with individuation. Correspondingly, Baudelaire, Rimbaud and Nerval, all visionary poets with a drug association, were redefined according to a hallucinogenic culture. But Kavan and J.G. Ballard had been living with this world as a reality from their youth, and were able to view a psychic substratum grow into a physical reality. The imagination grew briefly to be a social embodiment.

Kavan understandably had little or nothing in common with her British contemporaries, and it is probably only Leonora Carrington who approximates to Kavan's metamorphic, symbolist and imaginatively allegorical style of writing. Carrington gravitated to surrealism as a formative influence, and her *Down Below*, written at the time of her breakdown in Spain in 1943, explores a world in which alchemy, Lewis Carroll, surrealism and a hallucinated spectrum of theriomorphic images give voice to her madness. Her stories of the time, some of them written in a farmhouse at Saint-Martin-d'Ardèche, where she lived with Max Ernst, are full of animals who act as tutelary guides, horses and hyenas who have got on to the human wave-length. Kavan would have understood Carrington's maelstromic submergence in archetypes, and in her small, self-designed house in Hillsleigh Road, off Holland Park Avenue, surrounded by an abundance of exotic plants and conspiratorial mirrors, she inhabited her own imaginatively abundant microcosm. Her habit was not obtrusive to visitors, and addiction became apparent only on deeper acquaintance and at her own admission. But there are reports of her violent mood fluctuations, of her throwing a roast chicken across the dinner-table and then retiring to the bedroom to eat chocolates. She was solitary and inhabited the internalized visionary universe which has nothing to do with the dictates of literary fashion, for it is immutably modern. Inhabiting the outer regions of sanity, she intersected with what was peculiarly vital to her age: speed, drugs and the opening up of individuated psyche. She was a fine representative of that tradition of writers who work without remuneration or overt fame for the good of the imagination. In the richly textured surfaces of her writing she employs the sort of poetic vocabulary common to Virginia Woolf, Djuna Barnes and Anaïs Nin, but her vision supersedes all three, and her originality is incontestably compulsive.

In Kavan, a leopard will enter the room as a reality – she has that sort of direct contact with image. She monitors receptive invasion and selects the dominant archetype. It is all a matter of tuning. The visionary's excited neurological charge attracts by means of its resonance. Jung tells us that the archetype is based on inner and outer environment, and that the schematic model exists as a 'parallel arrangement of facts in time'.

> It looks [Jung writes] as if the collective character of the archetypes were not only inside the individual, but also outside, viz. in one's environment, as if sender and percipient were in the same psychic space, or in the same time in precognition cases. As in the psychic world there are no bodies moving through space, there is also no time. The archetypal world is 'eternal', i.e. outside time, and it is everywhere, as there is no space under psychic, that is archetypal, conditions. Where an archetype prevails, we can expect synchronistic phenomena, i.e. acausal correspondences, which consist in a parallel arrangement of facts in time.

Hyped up in the creative state, extraordinary intersections occur, 'as if sender and percipient were in the same psychic space', as Jung puts it, and as though the constellated image is dominant to the exclusion of all other psychic components. The writer has to sensitize as well as retrieve the image, that is to allow its sensory associations to deepen and connect. Again it is a matter of seeing. Kavan insights her subjective universe, and her intake of heroin was for her an adjustment to metabolic regularity rather than a removal from herself. The drug instated the subjective norm from which she functioned.

Writers get hooked on their own sense of reality and on the plurality of parallelism, and while in her early fiction (written under the name of Helen Ferguson) Kavan lacked the visionary dimension she developed in her later work, it is unlikely that this had to do with her increasing habit, for the drug had become her means of normalization rather in the way that Prozac has come to represent this for a new generation in search of a mood regulator. Kavan grew into her imaginary landscape, and as familiarity deepened, so the greater the risks she could entertain. She grew to live in the fictions she created. Like Kafka before her, she entered the labyrinth: 'I wondered where I was being taken. The place was colossal, the passages wound on and on. We passed the trapdoors of oubliettes, cells hacked out of the rock. The walls of these hutches were running with water, with some noisome exudation. Perilous steps led down to still deeper dungeons. We went through several pairs of huge doors, which the guards in front unlocked and the others slammed shut behind us.' (*Ice*)

Kavan's writing, like the drug she used, is a retreat into a secret interior. The work takes her into her own space. Her metaphors for the physical world generate extremes, nature grows to be still another alienating text, despite the descriptive sensuality with which she evokes a luxurious elemental universe. Her shadow side took her underground into subterranean mazes, corridors that lead to no conclusion, but that was also her gravitation to the deep silence of inner space. Sade, a prisoner for much of his adult life, was also attracted to conspiratorial silence, and the stimulus this provided both to his sexual fetishes and the setting of his fiction in castles and châteaux removed from the world.

When Kavan died, the Drugs Squad found an extraordinary supply of heroin stashed in her bathroom, a pharmaceutical hoard that the addict conceals for fear of being cut off from supply. There is always the phobic fear of being trapped somewhere, detained by the unexpected, or the obsessive worry that the drug may overnight cease to be manufactured. A compensatory measure must be found, and so the user learns to command larger or more regular prescriptions, or visits a number of doctors, or also scores on the street, and so a personal pharmaceutical archive is established. Elvis Presley had drugs prescribed for him by numerous doctors living in different states, and grew progressively and totally dependent on uppers and downers as well as a complex cross-reference of drugs for diverse deteriorative conditions connected with his colon and liver.

Anna Kavan's collection of short stories, *Julia and the Bazooka*, published posthumously, and some of which were written in the year preceding her death, manifest a more negative tunnel-vision than her earlier work, and the bazooka or needle becomes the explicit symbol of her alienation. Vertiginous panic, amnesia pockets, cryptomnesia, a dissociative personality and hypnopompic visions all infuse the writing, suggesting that she was becoming depersonalized by the drug. She often complained that she could feel nothing on an emotive level, and her long-term addiction had brought about significant and persistent changes in her biochemistry. At the end of her life, deprived of Dr Bluth's cushioning prescriptions, she was compelled to attend a drugs centre at regular periods on the demands of the Home Office. An exotically dressed Kavan (she owned forty different shades of lipstick, and had a wardrobe full of tastefully ostentatious clothes) was conveyed to and from the centre by taxis, a creature every bit as unusual as the leopard that entered one of her later stories, 'A Visit'.

Through her precognitive faculties Kavan clearly scented her own death, and in the pervasively autobiographical story 'Julia and the Bazooka', a harrowingly bilocated piece in which the protagonist undergoes numerous fantasy deaths (she is a young bride in a white dress as well as wreckage under an army blanket), she drives racing cars in accordance with Kavan's obsession with the latter and has permanently in her possession a bazooka or syringe, clearly Kavan's subjective portrait of components of herself. Kavan has the doctor say of the syringe to Julia:

> 'You've used it for years already and you're none the worse. In fact you'd be far worse off without it.' He trusts Julia, he knows she is not irresponsible, she does not increase the dosage too much or experiment with new drugs. It is ridiculous to say all drug addicts are alike, all liars, all vicious, all psychopaths or delinquents just out for kicks. He is sympathetic to Julia whose personality has been damaged by no love in childhood so that she can't make contact with people or feel at home in the world. In his opinion she is quite right to use the syringe, it is as essential to her as insulin to a diabetic. Without it she could not lead a normal existence, her life would be a shambles, but with its support she is conscientious and energetic, intelligent, friendly. She is most unlike the popular notion of a drug addict.

As an almost lifelong addict Kavan found it easier to continue her habit than to detoxify. She was functional within her own microcosm, and as such produced one of the most imaginatively original bodies of fiction in the English language. The nature of her work has led to marginalization by mainstream conservatism, but Kavan retains a considerable cult profile, and if times change to a more imaginative literary ethos her work will be acclaimed for its lyrical and visionary distinction.

Kavan is a perennial icon to outsiders. Durable writing, by which I mean an imaginative expression that is continuously anticipating the future, functions underground and is very often linked to a youth who are experimenting with fashionable street drugs. J.G. Ballard's hallucinated visions of the future intersected with a youth who had discovered the hallucinogenic properties of LSD, in the same way as Burroughs's work corresponded to a smack generation, and Kavan's work is textured into a whole synthesis of sensory experimentation, even if its cold climate is the product of heroin. Kavan's obsessive symbol is ice, or the big sleep. In 'Julia and the Bazooka' Julia has a vision of glacial depersonalization that corresponds to the emotional freeze induced by heroin: 'The cold is glacial, a glass dome of cold covers the globe. Icebergs tower high as mountains, furious blizzards swoop at each other like white wild beasts. All things are turning to ice in the mortal cold, and the cold has a face which sparkles with frost. It seems to be a face Julia knows, though she has forgotten whose face it is.'

Kavan's apocalyptic imagery and her sense of insighting universe are a long way from the anaesthetized regionalism that suffocates most late twentieth-century British fiction. But we are back to Lonely Street and Heartbreak Hotel. Who is waiting outside? The blue light flickers over the rain-washed street. There is a red curtain drawn in a window across the street. The outline of a woman undressing behind the curtain is visible to the solitary spectator. There is a public clock with broken hands propped up against a door. The hands have rusted. At any other time it would be late, but here it is always late and later. A car goes through, apparently without a driver and with no lights. The hotel has been standing in this sector ever since Elvis Presley first recorded 'Heartbreak Hotel' in 1956. The windows are blue glass behind boards. The aura of desolation is a moody, uncompromising one, and only particular people removed from their own time arrive at this mythic locus. Anna Kavan came and went. She stayed at the hotel for a time after one of her detoxifications. She got to know the maids in their blue suede shoes. She needed time and her private space in which to indulge her idiosyncrasies. She could walk outside directly into a hallucination. The street scene might have been written up in her head: no separation between inner and outer realities. Kavan in a blue wig and a ruby-sequinned dress.

Who do I see at the end of Lonely Street? He gets out of a glossy blue limousine driven by a young man with blond hair, and his arrival is graciously stylized. It is undoubtedly Jean Cocteau. A white scarf floats from his shoulders. His white shirt with the cuffs drawn over the sleeves of a Chanel jacket are part of his inimitable style. His face is characteristically emaciated, his long, bony fingers are studded with the dull blaze of jewels. He smokes a cigarette with the elegance of someone choreographing the escaped smoke. He has made flamboyance into a life-style which permeates his work, and his book *Opium* has contributed to the reputation he has for underground culture. Cocteau is a multifaceted Renaissance chameleon. He has come to Lonely Street because drugs have increased his isolation, and his gay coterie offer a surface reflection of his own histrionic temperament, but not consolation for the omnivorous overreach into all of the arts that have paradoxically won him both a reputation as an avant-garde proponent and a correspondingly disreputable name as a dilettante in all his pursuits. Lacking the volatile antagonism of the surrealists to bourgeois values, Cocteau has none the less made personal enemies of those who have opposed his own imaginative ideals. His support has always come from youth. His rebellion has been constant in its search for individuation at the expense of hypocritical morals. His unmanageable creative stimulus has resulted in the need to slow time. Opium for him is like stepping off an express train that is hurtling towards death. It takes him out of flux into timelessness. The drug connects with atemporal imagery.

Cocteau's addiction to opium began early in 1924 when, inconsolably traumatized by Raymond Radiguet's death, Cocteau went to stay in Monte Carlo for the Ballet Russe's winter season, and remained there with a group of friends which included a musicologist, Louis Laloy, who is presumed to have introduced Cocteau to opium. It is probable that Cocteau had been smoking opium intermittently for years, but his serious addiction grew out of the period immediately following Radiguet's death. 'My flight into opium is Freud's flight into sickness,' he wrote to Jacques Maritain, suggesting that the drug would become his epic admission to a parallel dimension. It is possible to see Proust's recourse to illness and the whole psychosomatic spectrum governing his retreat from life as an initiation into work and neurological subtext to self-awareness; and in a similar way, although on a much smaller canvas, some of Cocteau's best writing occurs in *Opium*, the book he wrote after his second attempt to detoxify in 1928. Like Proust, Cocteau had seen the necessity to evade life and to focus on imaginal interiority. Cocteau's life was hyper: he socialized with manic and ingratiating selectivity, and attached himself to the most illustrious of his contemporaries. He was also omnivorously prolific as a creative artist, and so opium became the anodyne to correct his mania. To the person who burns with creativity a decade is consumed like a month. There is never enough time, and the availability of the latter is contingent on finance, health and a variety of social intrusions that mediate between the artist and his work.

Cocteau's lifelong dialectic of paradoxes found both a resourceful and enervating locus in the drug he describes as a 'photographic negative of passion'. While the drug married past and future in recollective and anticipative sense associations, it suspended and killed libido. Opium may have mildly aphrodisiacal properties in the initial stages of dependency, but with continued use the penile nerves, especially those of the glans, become anaesthetized, and orgasm if it does occur is considerably retarded. The drug has a similarly depressing effect on the vaginal, vulval and rectal nerves in a woman. Cocteau writes of his temporary sexual debilitation in *Opium*, a theme that points to James Hillman's calling imaginal consciousness hermaphroditic, and as 'uniting masculine and feminine polarities, however they may be constellated at that moment'. Intense imaginal preoccupation dispenses with gender identity, and drugs can be another way of discovering dispersed sexuality and the libidinal simulacra we associate with hermaphroditic rather than polarized desire.

Cocteau was a prototypical icon for gay youth, and long before the media coverage given to a rock ethos young men copied his fashions, buying their ties at Charvet's and having their hair cut by Millat; they flirted with opium and acted as alumni of his beliefs and tastes. Cocteau asserted an unpublicized influence on the young as a proponent of drugs, and most notably as someone who perpetuated the legend of opium and the *poète maudit*. Baudelaire's *Les paradis artificiels*, together with the works of De Quincey, whom he pilfered, and Poe, whom he translated, invested the poet with an underground reputation and with the mystique of being someone who tempered his access to vision with liberal recourse to drugs. Nerval, Gautier, Rimbaud and Verlaine had perpetuated the myth as it was received by successive generations, and Wilde vividly portrayed the atmosphere of Limehouse opium dens in *The Picture of Dorian Gray*. There had been other casualties like the Austrian poet Georg Trakl, whose symbolist poetry bears much in common with Rimbaud's, and who was addicted to ether and morphine before committing suicide in 1914. The surrealists experimented with and used cocaine, and drugs had become identified with disaffected artists by the time Cocteau began his ineluctable liaison with opium.

Cocteau was too self-consciously a stylist ever to subscribe to Breton's notion of psychic automatism, but the painful attempts to detox that gave rise to the assemblage of sensory impressions and artistic reflection which comprise *Opium* are very much part of a literature of the hallucinated imagination. Cocteau was in and out of the drug, and like Michaux wrote directly from the experience, no matter how painful, and in *Opium* – of all his personal journals, with its accompanying disturbed drawings – he pursues a writing that touches the edge. More reflective than Michaux, and less dynamized by creating a psychobiography of the drug, Cocteau none the less in his enormously productive months at St-Cloud reflected deeply on areas of psychic geography which the drug had clearly sensitized into existence. His professed aim in taking opium was the evasion of the inevitability implied by life and death. 'Whatever one achieves in life,' he wrote, 'even love, happens in a fast train racing towards death. To smoke opium is to get out of the train while it is still moving. Its pursuit demands a concern with something other than life or death.'

That other is of course the interspace occupied by imaginal consciousness, the atemporal precinct in which the autonomy of images occurs. Living with inner space is like a potent fix. We go into it and come out changed, and in the process change the universe by the juxtaposed images we extract from the animated interior. 'The great images,' James Hillman tells us, 'are also the great passions; the places and caverns of memoria are also arenas of the inferno.' Drugs, like creativity, demand that the participant risks the fire. The visionary poet encounters a shamanic dismemberment, a psychophysical dispersal into altered states of consciousness, and on removal from trance experiences a corresponding regrouping of consciousness. The journey has been made. What is retrieved advances the work. It shines like a fistful of hot jewels.

Cocteau expressed the predicament of the man who lives his work totally and in the process is killed by it. He used opium as a means of attempting to resolve the paradox. 'Disgusted by literature, I wanted to go beyond it and live my work. And now I watch my work consuming me, adopting a life, while I die. Works invariably divide themselves into two: those which afford life, and those which kill.' Direct involvement with the work entails a dying into it, a risk that less committed writers are unable to confront, choosing instead a way of life in which a job mediates between them and their creative work. Cocteau, like all imaginative writers, professed a fierce commitment to his art. He lived it out to the full, the acquisitions, the wounds, the illnesses, habits and withdrawal agonies that his drug-dominated life demanded. He broke himself attempting to outrun time. Opium was his one means of slowing the manic orbit. 'The smoker's spirit moves without moving, like watered silk,' he wrote.

It is impossible not to see Cocteau's quest as heroic. He lived as though work was to be his singular redemption, and like all aesthetes his material was dependent on sensory associations and the corresponding exhaustion of his nerves that such a process entails. It was while withdrawing from opium at Saint-Cloud that he wrote his best-known novel, *Les enfants terribles,* within a manic period of three weeks. He attributed his inexhaustible creative fertility to magic, but in truth he worked to the detriment of his health, and his constant need to keep on proving his genius was to stay with him to the end of his life. He worked as though his entire *oeuvre* would be forgotten if he once let up. An ineluctable momentum pushed him towards scandal. 'My nature needs calm. My shadow side drives me towards scandal, like a somnambulist on the roof. The calm the drug induces used to protect me from a force which compels me to sit repentantly on a stool at a time when even the reading of a newspaper would destroy me.'

Cocteau's identification with youth, and his surrounding himself with a youthful entourage, in a way not so dissimilar from that of Andy Warhol, was at the roots of his gravitation towards scandal and rebellion. Opium was still another means of differentiating from bourgeois morality. Cocteau's hotel rooms, full of manuscripts, books, his personal mysteria, his drawing materials and make-up, were notoriously redolent of blue opium smoke. His complexion was often yellow, his figure emaciated, and he would disappear for days to purchase his supply. He was in search of dissociation and a return to childhood innocence. 'All children possess the magic power of being able to change themselves into what they wish. It is poets, in whom childhood is extended, who suffer terribly when they lose this gift. This is without doubt one of the reasons why poets use opium.'

The *puer aeternus* is of course an obsessive ideal with romantic poets. Imaginal consciousness is ageless; it is the biological process that wears out. Poetry is often an attempt to reverse the latter, and Cocteau in his ideas and choice of clothes tried to maintain the idea of permanent youth. His lovers were always younger men, and in his personal life he delighted in aggravating adults, or as he conceived it an older generation. Opium was incorporated into his inventory of symbols that subscribed to the *puer aeternus*. Cocteau inhabited a world of parapsychological rather than pathological phenomena, and while his work embodies mythic archetypes it does so on a more expository level than that of his visionary precedents and surrealist contemporaries. What he learnt from drugs was dissociation: 'The addict is surrounded by slopes. It is impossible to keep the spirit on the peaks. It is eleven o'clock at night; one looks at one's watch: it is five o'clock in the morning.'

And so we come back to the concept of missing time, those unaccountable pockets suggested by the experiences of UFO abductees, drug users, mystics, shamans and artists who go off somewhere else and return changed by their work. Entry into a parallel dimension is the cross-over into right hemispheric pressures. It sensitizes hallucination and generates the sort of hypnopompic visions which are signposts to a geography of the unconscious. I want more of the mystery in order to find my way to the interior. How many footprints did Dali, Ernst and Breton leave on that road? Millions, in their reorganization of how we see the universe.

It could be argued that Cocteau's films are more directly a product of his opomania than are his books. *Le sang d'un poète* and *Le testament d' Orphée*, both of which project an apotheosis of the artist as homosexual, are rich examples of what he called 'a kind of half-sleep in which I followed through my own labyrinth'. Tunnels, corridors, labyrinths, the way to the interior is a complex one inside an involuted maze. In *Le sang d'un poète*, the young man stripped to the waist plunges into the mirror and swims into the corridor of the Hôtel des Folies Dramatiques, where he negotiates an underworld of deliberate movements and pauses before each door voyeuristically to look through successive keyholes. In each of the rooms he discovers certain of Cocteau's salient obsessions. In the first, a young Mexican is shot twice to no effect and is able each time to rise in an act of indestructible nemesis. In the second room a girl is being taught to fly, and as a gesture of consummate defiance levitates and stares back at her earthed instructor. In the third room we see a hand in shadow on the wall insert an opium cone into his pipe. These dramatically juxtaposed visuals are closer to hallucinated imagery than the more consciously contrived symbols Cocteau employs in his poetry and fiction. They are the vocabulary of opium translated into film-frames. They are more directly the thought prints that flicker through imaginal consciousness.

Cocteau was forever undergoing unrealized cures, and his dependency on opium lasted for most of his adult life. Visitors to his various hotel rooms or small apartments would perceive Cocteau lying on his bed enveloped by an opium cloud. The drug had become much more than his identification with the lives of *poètes maudits*, it had become a stricture. 'I am living the predicament of people who, curious about poison, take some without understanding the danger,' he reflected. 'Impossible to backtrack. I am inhabiting death. It usually seeks out people in their homes. It will find me ensconced in its home.' It is related how, when Cocteau was forced to take part in the exodus of Paris at the time of the German occupation in 1940, he spent the morning prior to his departure searching for empty jam jars in which to store large quantities of fine opium, for his need had increased to thirty or forty pipes a day. He had come to integrate opium into his social and creative lives; the drug had become his ideated *monstre sacré*. But he was frightened and suffered the drug's hallucinatory terrors. 'After the waters of Paris clean water is too clean, too limpid – my mug frightens me and I'm sick: rheumatism, miseries, hideous fits of loneliness – unmentionable dreams.'

Cocteau seems never to have wanted properly to free himself of his habit. Opium added to the romantic Cocteau legend, and some of his recalcitrant defection from the adult world was in part supported by the drug. His creative world is a narcissistic one that rarely ventures outside his obsessive preoccupation with mythopoeticized youth and the classical myths he chose to incorporate into his thematic exploration of psyche. Essentially Cocteau tries to make legendary his own creative personae, and in the process goes against the grain of almost all prevailing schools of literature. He lived through the post-symbolist era of decadence, through Dada, surrealism, existentialism and the beginnings of the *nouveau roman,* but he took none of them on board. He formed his own avant garde, and refusing to admit to growing older remained a permanent icon to youth culture.

Cocteau belongs to Lonely Street by virtue of his drug habit and sexuality. He differs from Kavan in that he never sets out to create a literature about the hallucinated terrors attendant on a habit. Kavan's fiction is a progressive extension of her drug-alienated existence. At the Saint-Cloud clinic at the end of the twenties Cocteau wrote his novel *Les enfants terribles*, but the book does little to mirror his metabolic craving and psychic disturbance. On the contrary, he escapes into a world of childhood associations, whereas Kavan's writing becomes inalienable from heroin addiction. Both are writers who depended on a particular drug to counterbalance their adult lives, and both created an individualized body of imaginative work that allows it to transcend prevailing realist fashions. Moreover, both shared a love of dressing up for the invisible audience they called inspiration. Cocteau loved staging transvestite skits and costume became inseparable from his life-style, while the less gregarious Kavan dressed with exotic panache at home.

As in a still from one of his films, I shall leave Cocteau to disappear into the ruins of Heartbreak Hotel. In the first episode of *Le sang d'un poète*, a young man stands in front of a canvas on which he has painted a self-portrait. When the portrait's mouth begins to open, the artist attempts to erase the delusion with his hand, only to find that the mouth takes up its situation on his palm. When on the following day a female statue materializes, it comes alive and is afforded speech by the artist's attempt to transfer the mouth to the statue. Cocteau's animated images are the kinetic equivalent of his opium dreams. Inside Heartbreak Hotel he will go on projecting these. He will walk down corridors that telescope into more corridors, he will open doors into empty spaces in which clouds wobble through the sky. He will see a young man take out his eyes and drop them into a bowl of water, where they are metamorphosed into two green fish. He will see in another room Marilyn Monroe making up in a mirror that automatically takes up whatever angle she needs to reflect a plane of her face. The mirror flies away into a cloud. In another room a man is tapping a video cassette of dreams out of his head. The lights go out in the corridor. Cocteau is somewhere else. He lights a cigarette and walks into a wall of dark.

5

The connection between drugs, hallucination, breakdown and most expressions of twentieth-century art is an established truth. The long line of self-confessed addicts, extending from the Austrian poet Georg Trakl, someone who was remarkably influenced by Rimbaud, right through to William Burroughs and the Beat generation, has involved a pharmaceutical shift in seeing, and the excavation of an interior world as an opposing force to a predominantly material ethos. I take something, and I go somewhere else. I am a traveller by that distinction.

Georg Trakl, one of the great visionary lyric poets, died in a psychiatric ward in 1914 from an overdose of cocaine at the age of twenty-seven. In every characteristic embodying the bohemian decadence of the *poète maudit*, Trakl had trained as a pharmacist in Salzburg, and had from the age of fifteen taken to carrying a flask of chloroform with him and dipping his cigarettes into an opium solution. He additionally used morphine, veronal and cocaine. Deeply antisocial, pathologically wired to vision, incestuously attracted to his sister Grete, and living outside convention, Trakl was the prototypical rebel, one who burnt his life out prematurely, aspiring to ultimate vision. Trakl's neurotic sensibility and his agonized defiance of an increasingly bureaucratic century set him at odds with society in the manner of Rimbaud's youthful rebellion against capitalism. Trakl took up Rimbaud's credo that the poet makes himself a visionary through the process of 'a long systematic derangement of the senses', with committed vengeance. Fatally self-destructive, Trakl had as a child walked into a deep pond and kept on walking until he disappeared. It was only when his hat was seen floating on the surface that friends were alerted to the reality of the situation and dived in to rescue him. Arguably an early psychotic phenomenon, the incident was an indicator to much of Trakl's continuously obsessive behaviour, in which his detachment from the personal sanctity of life led to his recklessly testing the frontiers of death. Possessed of a Baudelairean fascination with evil, Trakl in his poetry explores a complex inner world of sexual guilt, hallucinated reality, mythic archetypes, and turns inwards towards the atavistically primal as a means of the poet avenging himself on a society with which he was acutely uncomfortable. Something of the momentous build-up to the European war in 1914, a climate that proved to be the prevailingly portentous *Zeitgeist* for Trakl's generation, leaked into the poet's psyche right from the beginnings of his work as an Expressionist.

Trakl's poetry works on the edge of disintegration, the absolute clarity of its images coloured by the apprehensive cataclysm that is always impending, be it personal breakdown or universal catastrophe. For Trakl there was no resolution to inner torment through the projective means of writing poetry, for one set of complexes is simply replaced by another. The poet does not gain from the poem; that privilege is delegated to the reader. Trakl's poetry has a remorseless circularity: the poet is unable to break the circuit of psychic anguish, which affords it its compelling power and correspondingly its death-trap mechanism to the poet. Unable to escape his psychosexual obsessions, Trakl attempted to find relief in drugs, or in heavy drinking, and his anguished, taciturn, unsociable sensibility presented itself to the inner trajectory.

In his hallucinated, intensely subjective drug-world Trakl was able to confront his shadow and establish discourse with the poetic underworld. Cocaine lined him into a state of temporary euphoria, and veronal served as a downer. In a letter written by Frank Zeis (an acquaintance of Trakl's) to a friend in 1913, Zeis describes the poet as 'A dear person, silent, reserved, shy, entirely turned inward. Looks strong, powerful, but at the same time sensitive, sick. Has hallucinations, and raves.' We learn additionally from this letter of Trakl's dislike of eye contact, and how when he travelled by train he would stand in the corridor rather than risk being scrutinized by a stranger. Trakl was also pathologically frightened of any inadvertent physical contact with strangers, and protected himself from being brushed by a shoulder in the street or jostled in a crowd. He disliked large cities and would sometimes sleep out in the woods or countryside surrounding Innsbruck. He shared with Rimbaud a desire to retain a state of visionary innocence, one that was uncorrupted by adult and societal machinations. And like Rimbaud, he was happiest on the road, communing with the animated Pan-informed spirit of nature. Part of Trakl's habit owed its origins to his reluctance to accept responsibility for living. He felt unable to commit himself to life and, constantly delaying the process, reverted psychologically to states supported by primal, mythic consciousness. Drugs and poetry formed an inseparable symbiosis for him, for both allowed him access to the autonomy of visionary states. Trakl belonged to a tradition of writers, often associated with drugs, who, turning away from the created world with its complex ideological systems, set out to invent an individualized microcosm, one that owed its origins to the imagination. On the inner dimension everything is possible, the poet in his juxtaposition of images becomes the god of imaginal consciousness. In a letter to his patron and friend, Ludwig von Ficker, Trakl in referring to his sister's marital problems, and to his own state of inner fragmentation, writes: 'I no longer know in from out. It is such an indescribable disaster when one's world breaks apart. Oh my God, what a judgement has broken over me. Tell me that I must have the power to live on and to act truthfully. Tell me that I'm not insane. A stony darkness has broken in. Oh my friend, how small and unhappy I have become.'

Trakl, who worked intermittently as a pharmacist in Salzburg, until exposure to the public proved too much for his fragile nervous sensibility, was constantly in need of money to finance his immoderate habits. Unsuited to a profession, and entirely preoccupied by inner events, Trakl was helped by Ludwig von Ficker, who was the first to see the poet's genius, and indirectly by Ludwig Wittgenstein, who wishing to give away some of his large paternal inheritance to indigent Austrian artists, settled money on Rilke, the painter Oskar Kokoschka, and Trakl. Trakl was never to benefit from this annuity, and on the one occasion he went to the bank accompanied by Ficker, he ran out of the building in a state of panic, signally unable to cope with the money made available for his disposal. And like Rimbaud's, his life was founded on financial insecurity. His poetry embraced a world in which money played no part, and in his gravitation towards ontological awareness, Trakl looked to a state of pure essence as the signifying state of poetry. It is his uncompromising defection from reality which affords his poetry its sense of angular defiance. Trakl turned his back on the idea of civilization, he walked out on all conventional orders, located his sexual energies in his sister (who was also to kill herself), and generated a poetry in which colour, synaesthesia and image rather than symbol were the imaginal dominants.

Trakl once described his short life as involving 'days of delirious drunkenness and criminal melancholy', and he was known to consume alcohol until he dropped; and living totally through the identity of a poet, he may well have used hard drugs in order to feel less the unnerving lapse in inspiration at times when he was not writing. Periods of disattunement from the imagination are less noticeable to writers who pursue other employment, but to those who live out the reality of their imaginative calling guilt and anxiety feature strongly in periods of dormant creativity. Trakl needed to live in the charge of his writing, and drugs provided a compensatory stimulus for the periods when there was nothing else around. There was also the sense of psychophysical experimentation involved in using drugs to achieve altered states of mind. Trakl was hard on himself in ways that again bear similarities to Rimbaud, both poets seeming to care little for personal comfort, and both being equally prepared to undergo the shaman's metaphorical death in order to realize vision. Trakl is known to have lapsed into unconsciousness in the snow, and to have spent the night in those sub-zero conditions and survived. The degree of his psychic anguish called for a corresponding chemical corrective, and there are no indications that Trakl ever looked to depathologize his symptoms by consultation. He prescribed for himself, bought drugs illicitly, and used his pathology as the energy-drive behind his work.

Something of the state of Trakl's disappointment with life, in the sense of imaginative aspiration seldom finding its counterpart in reality, is evidenced in a letter Trakl wrote to Karl Heinrich in the year preceding his death: 'I do not have easy days at home now and I drift between fever and helplessness in sunny rooms where it is unspeakably cold. Strange shudders of transformation, bodily experienced to the point of unbearability; visions of mysteries until the certainty of having died; ecstasies to the point of stony petrifaction; and a continuation of dreaming sad dreams.'

Trakl was in every way dissociated from his body. He saw the latter as a source of putrefaction, and as a vessel too opaque for the transparency of his mind. He inherited Baudelaire's preoccupation with disease and sexual guilt, and like so many drug users pursued a largely asexual existence in which heightened nervous stimulus compensated for lack of sexual sublimation. The anima figure in Trakl's work is always the sister, who likewise experimented with drugs, and who much to Trakl's anguish ended up marrying the much older Arthur Langen, a Berlin journalist, before shooting herself through the head in Berlin, three years after her brother's suicide. There is of course a case to be made for incest being in some way responsible for both deaths, and as a contributing source to Trakl's unrenounced habit. Trakl used liberal amounts of veronal in order to assist sleep, and on one occasion attempted to kill himself with this drug, suffering the unpleasant toxic discomforts of veronal poisoning. He took the cult of the sacrificial poet, the shaman readily advancing his own ritual dismemberment, further than Rimbaud, for the latter was without Trakl's inexorably morbid sensibility, and was possessed of a healthy disrespect for an art which he seems to have known in advance would fail him. Rimbaud was adventurously resilient and was able to walk away from the fire he had lit, whereas Trakl wished only to be consumed by his singular vision. The youthful psychopathologies informing the work of both poets point to remarkable similarities in their concerns with image, and colour as an associative synaesthetic state. Rimbaud's dimensions are wider and more innovative than Trakl's obsessively narrowed field of subjective concerns, but both poets apprehended the liberation of the unconscious, which had begun effectively with Lautréamont's *Maldoror* in 1870, and which was to become increasingly the imaginal province of twentieth-century psychology. Trakl dips both his feet into the image-pool, whereas Rimbaud dived to the bottom in order to retrieve marvels.

Trakl used drugs indiscriminately to alter his state of consciousness, and not experimentally with the idea of creating out of the process. His poetry was of course an extension of his pharmaceutical input, but only accidentally. It was living that proved unbearable, and part of the terror the poet experienced in the real world is transferred to the menace that inhabits his poetry, the wolves, dark strangers, complementary selves which show up again and again in his visionary landscapes. Trakl is essentially a poet of autumn: he evokes decay, the rotting fruit, the wound as it occurs in the earth and in his psyche. His poems are invariably crepuscular or nocturnal in their settings, and they use silence as an atmospheric mechanism to the exclusion of all other states. One can feel Trakl slipping into inner space and waiting for a familiar interior landscape to claim him in the way one anticipates the effects of a drug coming on before the chemical release takes full effect. Trakl's entry-point into the poem is ambivalently charged, for the space offers him redemptive vision as well as disillusionment in that the return journey will resituate him in a field of trauma.

Trakl established a real antipathy for Salzburg and Vienna, the two big cities in which he had working and living experience. Most drugs create alterating paranoid claustrophobic or agoraphobic symptoms, and Trakl manifests evidence of both disturbances in his life and poetry. His tone is one of shutting all the doors in order to give voice to his agony. Unable as he was to sing of the pain like a broken, drug-wrecked Billie Holiday or Judy Garland, his communication came through the tone of his compellingly hermetic poetry. Like all obsessives, Trakl had essentially one poem and one voice, and he returned to this specific psychic precinct again and again. His is a poetry that attempts to locate a mythopoetic state of innocence, but it is the acknowledgement that this condition has no place in the real world which lends Trakl's poetry its inimitably elegiac properties. He carries loss in his hands like his sister's miscarried child and is constantly agonized by the realization that poems have no meaning in the ordering of the external universe. Unable to turn away from his creative source, he obstinately returns in search of the help which he knows in advance will be denied him.

His habit complied to a similar pattern. Under drugs, and rather like writing poetry, he could monitor the hallucinated archetypes of his inner world, he could acquaint himself with the contents of his unconscious, but it was an individualized, subjective world that would not carry over into reality. Trakl's gravitation towards suicide was in direct proportion to the rift he experienced between inner and outer realities. Trakl's work was done in secret, and inner riches have no place in the system of material currency. Big events occurred in the poet's psychological cosmos: 'Shepherds buried the sun in the barren woods./ A fisherman/ Pulled in the moon in a thin net from the freezing pond.' If the medical diagnosis of *dementia praecox,* or schizophrenia, were correct in its application to Trakl in his last weeks in a military mental hospital, prior to his suicide, then the condition was probably aggravated by the poet's indiscriminately liberal use of drugs.

It is suitably apocalyptic in connotations that Trakl should have worked in 1911–12 as a dispenser in the White Angel, one of Salzburg's oldest pharmacies and the place of his apprenticeship. Trakl undoubtedly stole drugs in his innumerable short-lived periods of employment as a dispenser, for he had little money with which to accommodate his habit. He turned in on extreme psychological states, attempting to validate the myth of the poet as madman, as he who differs by virtue of access to the animated imagination. Drugs for Trakl were a way of taking him further out on that committed trajectory, and they were also his source of identity amongst friends. Most committed poets since the time of Baudelaire have felt a sense of social exile, of not belonging to the corporate ethos, and have often chosen to pronounce their difference by cultivating the role of self-immolative victim. Denied the support structure that surrounded the shaman's tribal consciousness, the poet in taking up a continued discourse with the imagination is often the unpronounced shaman defiantly retaliating by opening the wound within himself. Trakl's relatively provincial world of Innsbruck and Salzburg had neither time nor place for such a voice. And for the poet informed by universal ideals, caught up in the concrete maze of big cities, and forced to keep alive in an unsympathetic social environment, the psychic role of being an unliberated shaman, nurtured by peyote rites, has taken the inverted route of neurotic drug dependence, or else pathological symptoms which in turn lead to breakdown.

It would be discouraging to see Trakl as simply another casualty in the line of uncompromising *poètes maudits*. His worldly aspirations were few: he made an application to be a pharmacist in Borneo, but rather with the same impractical resources that Rimbaud brought to his application to join the US Navy; he concerned himself with his sister's unhappy marriage and with the immediate lives of his small circle of friends. Beyond that he showed little ambition with regard to material advancement. He was active for short periods with the military, and entered into service in the 1914 war with a sense of spiritual elation, perhaps seeing in it a means of escaping the distaste he felt for pedestrian life. His highly strung nerves were quickly to snap at the sight of carnal atrocities, and it was partly the ordeal of looking after the mutilated without adequate medicines at his disposal which precipitated his suicide. Trakl's poetry had anticipated apocalyptic catastrophe on an inner plane, but he was little physically qualified to deal with the reality.

Trakl lived his life acquainting himself with death. He once remarked to his friend, Theodor Däubler: 'We fall into an inapprehensible darkness. How could dying, the moment which leads to eternity, ever be short?' And his poetry leans against that question, it talks into the psychic space he imagined to be death. There is something to be learnt of Trakl's morbid autophobia in the psychological writings of Alfred Adler, a contemporary of Trakl's, who suggested: 'The realization of somatic inferiority by the individual becomes a permanent impelling force for the development of his psyche.' Trakl, whose letters are full of self-indictments as to the decaying organism of his body, chose to neglect the physical and to deepen psyche. His inner world is bright with illumination, in contrast to the shadow with which he surrounded his body. Drugs and alcohol were a means of damaging the physical, and Rimbaud, again in relation to characteristics shared with Trakl, appears also to have had little care for his body and to have regarded it as inferior to mind. Both poets used the body as a source of psychophysical experimentation.

But there is a real and significant difference between the lives of those who use drugs and those who do not. This has to do with the subjective notation of dependency and how this affects social interaction, as well as contributing to the inner absorption surrounding the user's preoccupation with chemical changes brought about by drugs. There is no forgetting a need. Wherever you are and whatever you are doing, it is uppermost in consciousness. Like Anna Kavan, Trakl has left no personal journal describing his dependency, and both writers inhabited a personalized microcosm of creativity, their chemicalized imbalance registering in their work, their drug obsession being reflected in the obsessive nature of their narrow, but universally orientated themes. It seems consistent that obsessive writing deepens rather than expands, it needs the reassurance of familiar images in the way the metabolism feeds on the necessary drug. It is interesting to note that drugs seem never to have radically expanded Trakl's image repertoire; his imaginal universe is predictably stable, and I think this is so because it provided him with a point of refuge. The same bleak landscape inhabited by ruins, desolate in its autumnal decay, peopled by the anima figure of a sister or angel, or the animus persona of a shepherd, and embodying the colours blue, red, purple, silver and black, is the unchanging matrix in which the poem is situated. Trakl's poetry is coloured by hallucination, but more as a natural way of seeing rather than as an artificially induced state. And it is a world that excludes people: Trakl's poetry is essentially about himself and the other, and the psychic anguish generated by his pervading mood of disquiet. He was known to sit in company for hours and not say a word, and then to make a declaratively lateral statement totally disconnected from the issues being discussed.

In a letter to Irene Amtmann, Trakl comments on the long walks he took, partly walking out on himself, as well as setting up the inner rhythm to communicate with the world around him: 'It seems to me that I wander around daily like a vagabond, at times in the forests which are already turning red and where marksmen harass the wild life to death, or I explore disconsolate streets in the bleak areas of town, or simply lounge around Salzach and watch the seagulls. . . . Forgive this madman who would rather slip into a peasant's skin than make verses in the sweat of his face.'

Trakl and Rimbaud both identified with the earthy ideal of the peasant, and Trakl, rather like the nervous deer who slip fluently in and out of his poetry, preferred to hide in the woods and plot his creative revenge on the world. He was charged by elemental contact. He possessed what Jung has called an 'obedience to awareness', and in his earth orientation he is closer to shamanic vision, and the often painful awakening of the mythic imagination, than to a poetry involving a register of the modern city. He resists the civilized topos which Baudelaire had made the condition of the new poetry. And like the shaman Trakl engages with chaos in the attempt to re-establish a vocabulary that interrelates all animate things.

Something of the implosive turbulence of the shamanic quest is apparent in all of Trakl's writings. His was a process of excavating the interior, and something of his inexorable hold on his work (he never loses power over the constituents of his poem) has to do with the shaman's ability to arrest the inchoate and transform it into reconstituted form. Habitual ways of seeing and conceiving the world break down under shamanic ritual, and access is afforded to the visionary *mysterium*. Trakl's poetry is very much about this ordering process, the journey through chaos towards mystic realization. In most cultures the shaman is assisted in his inner journey by the use of ceremonial drugs, and the twentieth-century poet divorced from this tribal context has been left to prescribe for himself in the attempt to resacralize vision.

The Heartbreak Hotel that Trakl came to eventually was a military asylum. In March 1914 his sister had a miscarriage accompanied by extraordinarily vehement bleeding, and Trakl hurried to Berlin to offer her emotional support. It seems more than probable that they shared a drug dependency, and that the incestuous nature of their relationship brought strain to bear on Grete's marriage. Grete, who was an accomplished musician, would play her brother Schubert sonatas on the piano, and she would undoubtedly have shared the perverse decadence that led Trakl to dip his cigarettes into an opium solution. Grete seems to have suffered the same financial insecurity as her brother, and Trakl felt guilt at being unable to provide for her, despite the fact she was married. By August of that year, Austria had declared war on Serbia, and Trakl was appointed lieutenant in the Innsbruck brigade of the Army Medical Corps. The idea of a paranoid, neurotic junkie, with a red carnation in his cap, boarding a cattle-train for Poland is in itself a sufficient condemnation of the military independent of the suicide it provoked.

Trakl, who was not even a regularly practising pharmacist in civilian life, and whose behaviour had consistently manifested the delusional symptoms at the heart of his poetry, found himself moved in a field-hospital unit to Galacia, a province in Poland. It was at Grodek, a scene commemorated in one of his last poems, that Trakl's unit was subject to a bloody defeat, and the atrociously unrelieved suffering of the wounded, ninety of whom were placed in a barn under Trakl's care, and the dementia of those driven mad by shock and the appalling carnage they had witnessed, were the catalogue of victims presented to his medical authority. Outside of the barn, there was a line of partisans and deserters hanging from the trees. As we know it, Trakl ran out of the barn towards the trees and attempted to shoot himself in the head before being disarmed by another soldier. Two weeks later, and with the fear of being court-martialled for 'cowardice in the face of the enemy', Trakl, who had managed to conceal a quantity of drugs on his person, was transported to a garrison hospital in Cracow. It appears that the military already had reservations about Trakl's mental health, for his poetry had been scrutinized by the authorities censoring mail, and the question of madness seems to have been raised. Trakl was placed in a cell with bars over the window, a constricted space he had to share with a lieutenant suffering from delirium tremens. He was officially under psychiatric observation, wore prison clothes, and his condition was exacerbated by the cacophonic shrieks of the insane. He was visited inside by Ludwig von Ficker, who tried hard to intervene for Trakl's release, fearing that his friend's depressed condition would result in intentional death. Trakl communicated with Ficker from the hospital, sending him small revisions to poems, and requesting that in the event of his death his sister should benefit monetarily from his assets. Trakl died of a large overdose of cocaine early in the morning of 3 November 1914, bringing his short, tormented life to an abrupt conclusion.

Trakl's place in the pantheon of *poètes maudits* was assured by his life rather than his death. He committed himself to the retrieval of imaginative vision, and lived with all the material vulnerability that such a pursuit entails. It is interesting to quote one of the psychiatric reports made on Trakl during his enforced stay at Cracow, for it emphasizes delusional aspects of Trakl's inner world, paranoid fictions which, while they fed his poetic imagination, were difficult to reconcile with functional living. The psychiatric report reads:

> From time to time since his childhood he has had visual hallucinations. It seems to him that a man with a drawn knife stands behind his back. From twelve to twenty-four years of age, he saw no such apparitions. For three years now he has again been suffering from these optical illusions and, moreover, he often hears bells ringing. He did not believe that his father was his own, but rather imagined that he descends from a cardinal and that in the future he will become a great man.

A medically conclusive diagnosis of pathological schizophrenia, which at the time was considered incurably deteriorative, would possibly have led to Trakl's confinement. The poet feared prolonged detainment as much as he did returning to the war. And here there is a problem over the signifiers of language. Visual and auditory hallucinations are the currency of imaginative art, but if they are transferred to a confessional mode, if they are described as existing independent of their creative function, they are considered pathological, and comprise behavioural aberrations that come under the province of psychiatric scrunity. Trakl in describing his inner states would have used the imagistic language of his poetry, he would not have separated inner from outer awareness, and to a psychiatrist unresponsive to the creative image-pool his language would appear to have symptomatized *dementia praecox*. The report also emphasized by the use of quotation marks the anomaly that the patient 'wrote poetry'. Abnormality was implied by the latter occupation, a form of expression that must have appeared additionally antipathetic to the military. Soldiers are supposed to be concerned with immediate reality and not its transformation into a parallel frequency. Trakl's poetic verbalization would have been seen as synonymous with schizophrenic speech. Trakl's symptoms would have been related to organic pathology.

Around the time that Trakl was minting his hallucinated lyrics, Marcel Proust had virtually confined himself to the voluntary invalidism of someone constricted to a life spent in bed. Proust, with his highly strung neurotic sensibility, the conditioner of his psychosomatic asthma, was also one addicted in large parts to the substances he took to relieve nervous crises.

At the heart of Proust's work, and few writers have afforded a more suprasensible architecture to inner space, extending sense associations to a neural cosmography in which place and time are retrieved with an almost disquieting exactitude, lies an imbalance which is respiratorial, and by virtue of that flaw chemicalized, adjusted, individual by way of defect. Asthma, orthopnoea, cardiac spasms, asphyxiation, Proust's diagnoses or misdiagnoses describe also a state which for him represented imaginative creativity. 'My attacks give no warning,' he wrote to Robert de Montesquiou. 'I might find myself that very day incapable of getting out of bed, or even speaking, in the throes of asphyxiations as unbearable for you as for me, and with a fever amounting almost to delirium.'

Proust's intake of drugs centred upon uppers and downers: caffeine for use as a stimulant and veronal as a sedative. I stress this aspect of Proust's life, for his dependency on drugs, either as a means psychologically to allaying an incipient asthma crisis or to reactivating a chemistry dulled by sedation, is powerfully reflected in his work. Contraction and dilation. The former involved Proust in a process of endless visual retrieval, and the excavation of psychic states with their corresponding experiential values accounts for the minutiae of psychological perception which is inseparable from his genius. Correspondingly, dilation, the euphoria that often occurs after a severe nervous crisis, the outbreath acquiring expansion after constricting panic, has much to do with the escalating spiral of Proust's syntax. His breath-flow is one in which image resonates against image, and almost always in a visual sense, so that the evocation of colour may lead from the recollection of a flower to a painting, to a sunset, to a dress, to the evaluation of a character trait in which all these qualities are combined. And it is the imagination that creates these interworlds for Proust. Illness and chemical imbalance made him restructure the world with so omnivorous an eye for detail that the barriers between imagined and real no longer existed.

Proust's letters invariably contain two conditions: 'I have been so ill, I am still so ill.' He was given little respite from respiratory crises, and like all those who anticipate the spasmic trauma of hyperventilation, or in Proust's case a breathlessness that approximated to asphyxia, he tried desperately to pre-empt the attacks by the use of drugs. And as a condition of psychological terror, he was quick to translate anxiety into physiological terms. 'For I'm very much afraid that these incessant attacks have destroyed something in my organism which will never be able to recover.'

In his biography of Proust, Ronald Hayman describes the effects of the Legras powders with which Proust incessantly fumigated. Hayman writes:

> He may have been aware the powders were addictive–sometimes he made efforts to stop 'smoking'–but he didn't realize that in a bedroom ventilated only by the draught from the chimney, the carbon monoxide produced from burning the powders and the wood could have helped to cause the malaise he progressively suffered – headaches, nausea, exhaustion, weakness of vision and changes in the function of his central nervous system. The powders contained atropine and byoscyamine,

which relieved the asthma by dilating and drying the bronchial tree, but also tended to blur the vision by dilating the pupils, and it could have contributed to the weakness, giddiness, cardiac palpitation and the disturbance of speech and gait he was later to suffer.

If there is a homogeneous drug literature, and I am thinking of the opium dependency in the lives of Coleridge, Baudelaire and Cocteau, the profligate use of hallucinogens by Rimbaud and Michaux, Artaud's involvement with a variety of drugs from opium to heroin, the heroin need inherent in the lives of Anna Kavan and William Burroughs, then Proust is part of that chemical chain, his obsession with alleviants amounting almost to an oral fixation. Once reality becomes an invasive threat, the compensation is artificiality, the adjustment of the metabolism to a tempo that seems proportionate to imaginative volume.

Proust's anxiety looked for stopping-off points in places constellated by memory, childhood, paintings, architecture, an individual flourish of dress, and the effect of this richly textured mosaic is to show us the outer surface of his nervous complexity. Information stored in the memory cells, tonal propensities, meditations on nature and art, a whole storage system which had been withheld, spiral into a reflective magnitude, a release contingent on imbalance and the creative condition on which they meet the world. Proust is in part describing the unconscious – the dark, green pool in which images flicker or browse murkily like fish. And writing as he did, under extreme paucity of light, the source generated by a green-shaded lamp, Proust with his curtains drawn on the seasons, and not dating his letters for fear of the advancing years, lived in the half-light, the intermediary stage between the unconscious and its realization through writing, transmission on to the white glare of the page.

'And my life is so bizarre and lamentable that whenever I talk about it I give the impression of apologizing', he wrote to Max Daireaux. The combination of genius and its modification through the chemical permutations of drugs created in Proust the role of a messenger between worlds. How well he would have understood Rilke's poem 'Orpheus, Eurydice and Hermes' with the thin god in the cobalt cloak eating up the road as he made rapid strides out of the underworld. What Proust ate up, with an insatiable rapacity, was memory. Unable to detach himself from his past, he made the re-creation of it into a timeless present. The mobility he had achieved in relation to inner space was in contrast to his inert, valetudinarian body. 'I go out once a month for an hour, and afterwards, quite apart from attacks of asthma, have to spend a week in bed.'

The situation appeared intolerable. Constant palpitations made Proust fear a cardiac condition, but he did little to moderate his intake of the caffeine which was a contributing factor to his disquieting tachycardia. Around this time, September 1904, he considered undergoing psychotherapeutic treatment in a clinic, a notion to which he was to return again and again, without the motivation to put the theory into practice. Like most creative people, he preferred to live with the idea of his illness and translate physical malfunction into imaginative gain. Proust who, in his writing, lived outside time, occupying a space in imaginal consciousness, nevertheless regarded his body as a source of anguished, temporal decay, a mechanism involved in an irreversible catabasis punctuated by violent attacks of asphyxia. And if his life was a preparation for imminent death, its quality was heightened as a consequence.

Few writers have evoked the joy of living as a transcendental counterpart to death in the manner that Proust was to do in his reflectively experienced novel. If Proust appears to live at the centre of a diamond, out of which he cannot break, the study of his life within those refractive interfaces is the story of someone who, in Rilke's phrase, subscribes to the notion 'Who speaks of winning: surviving is all.'

Constantly contracted in his effort to meet the world, his breathing irregular, his diaphragm tensed to anticipate the muscular spasm, Proust approached health with suspicion. If in terms of yoga breath represents a gift independent of man, a fluency which lives him, Proust turned respiration into a conscious, embattled process.

In the attempt to ward off asthmatic convulsions Proust smoked Espic cigarettes and burned medicated powders by his bedside.

Hypochondria, microphobia, a deeply ingrained agoraphobia – Proust would travel only by a car which collected him – all combined to establish a reverse process of living. He set himself visually and emotionally to retrieve the past, and to imagine the present as a continuity of disjunctive time. An intensified moment in which the word substituted for distress. In his writing Proust aims to establish the physical expansion that his body could never meet. It is little wonder that his novel is a house of images built to encompass the universe. Hayman tells us that to send himself to sleep Proust used a combination of Trional, Valerian and Amyl. 'Trional was a hypnotic drug consisting of an ethyl sulphone. Valerian, a herbal sedative, had been popular throughout the nineteenth century. Amyl was a tertiary amyl alcohol currently in use as a sedative.'

I write this on an afternoon when snow shuts in the world, reduces everything to a prismatic dazzle. That leopard-spotted thrush is suddenly too huge, too articulate. Its jewelled brown eyes emphasize the separation of consciousness between myself and it. And it expands, grows to the actual size of a leopard, is huge, predatory and menacing under a violet sun. And suddenly I am reminded of how long Lorazepam asserted a tyranny over my metabolism. On bad days, shapes still change dramatically with such a protean, hallucinated content that I have to unlearn seeing and retreat into the interior. And where am I inside? I see myself running towards a huge mirror with the leopard-sized thrush struggling in my arms.

In a letter Proust wrote to his mother sometime in 1905, his condition of stress was such that he mentions the possibility of using heroin to alleviate the situation. I quote the letter in full:

> Please don't fail to have someone in this evening. Although I'm a thousand times less in pain, I'm naturally spending a far worse day than yesterday, as so far it's been impossible to rest lying down, even without going to sleep, and I'm fumigating all the time. As a precautionary measure you might get some heroin on the off-chance, although I'm absolutely determined not to take any. But one can't tell what might happen with these attacks, that are so unlike what I've been used to. So it

would be much better to be prepared than to have to wake up a chemist tonight.

I feel better at the moment. I hope this rain will put me in better condition. Please get the heroin in any case, just for safety's sake.

While she was alive, Proust used his mother as a confidante in matters pertaining to his asthmatic condition. He monitored his crises with a diaristic and self-diagnostic obsession. By projecting his fears on to her, he was able to find comfort in diminishing the sense of isolation that comes about through nervous terror. It is possible to reach a state in which a white tiger sits in one's head, showing its blue eyes, threatening one with nervous paralysis should it move a step forward, or flex a muscle lazily in sleep. Proust shared each intimate detail of his drug habit with his mother:

> Back home at 11 p.m. precisely. Felt rather oppressed (in spite of several Espics during the day), had a fumigation. It was my first time alone, so it all took ages. Went to bed at a quarter past twelve, got up again, back in bed at half past (time by the clock in your boudoir), chest tight in spite of fumigation, took two capsules of amyl. Sleep came quickly. 5.30 a.m. awakened by oppression or at least with oppression, indeed with rather severe panting. Got up and had an energetic fumigation with Escouflaire and Legras powders . . . (Letter 2 September? 1896)

There was a vicious trap involved here. In order to demand attention from his mother, Proust considered he had to be ill. It was a mode of behaviour that was expected of him. His mother would not have recognized a healthy son, and to be the latter would have involved letting go of the past which was so vital to his work, and relinquishing hold on the obsessively fetishistic world his imagination had come to inhabit. Proust stored everything. The most complex, diverse and elusive sense-associations were activated through writing to a holistic synaesthesia. Marcel would have had time stand still, only the physical effort involved in writing demanded that he enter the temporal flux, that journey in which we grow physically old as a contradiction to the timelessness of inner space.

Cardiac spasms and angina pectoris, and a serious undermining of the central nervous system, owing to his too liberal use of opium-based anti-asthma powders, were only some of the disquieting symptoms that kept Proust confined to bed, unwilling to take any form of exercise, and living as the horrified annotator of his own dissolution. 'The torment of the neurasthenic is out of all proportion to the gravity of its cause,' he noted. And as early as 1905, Proust felt that his body could not survive the intensity of his panic-convulsions. While caffeine, taken in tablet form, relaxed his breathing, it also made his arms and legs shake if he attempted physical exertion. His asthma attacks, which were accentuated by paroxysms induced by drug poisoning, could last for anything up to twenty-four hours. At such times he suffered from a condition called orthopnoea, in which the person can breathe only by maintaining a standing posture.

Proust's confidence that he would outlive his condition by writing, and play tricks on respiratorial dysfunction by a retreat to the interior, is amongst the great heroic postures in literature. Underlying his creative furore was the private myth that he would be well one day, and that life would commence without reference to an injurious past. Hadn't he also a right to live? But illness was inextricably linked to his creative source, so much so that the realized expansion of time granted to an invalid would correspondingly represent the allocation of undisturbed hours in which to write. And to enforce his reclusion, Proust inverted night and day, his day not beginning until three or four in the afternoon, and his writing hours occupying the night, with occasional visits to restaurants or friends occupying the hours between ten and midnight. The eccentricity of his life freed him from the pressures of social obligations, and the night as it was for Novalis and Rilke became for Proust a black diamond, a depth invested with absolute clarity and silence, a passage which had to be accompanied by a story – an accompanying inner voice which grew to be *A la recherche du temps perdu*.

Proust's doctors were as numerous as the prescriptions given him. They included Dr Pierre Merklen, who in 1904 referred Proust to the clinic of Dr Paul Dubois in Berne. There was Dr Henri Vaquez, who in 1902 diagnosed Proust's tachycardia as nervous and not cardiogenic in origin; Dr Widmer, with whom Proust took a rest cure at Valmont in 1905; and Dr Maurice Bize, who remained Proust's general practitioner and who advocated injections of camphorated alcohol to help relieve congestion of the chest.

What a man does in his private hours, with only himself as witness to the accompanying act, can be perversely self-destructive. There is a complicitous pact in this, the notion of duality. Whatever miscalculated doses of drugs Proust took in his dressing-room at 102 Boulevard Haussmann involved the element of clandestinity by which he lived. Answerable as he made himself to his mother, even after her death, his manner oscillated between revenge for the infantilism she had instated in him and a constant desire to re-create her through his writing. The misuse of drugs was one way of defying her; so too was his perverse decision to furnish the male brothel he owned during the First World War years with his parents' furniture. Jean Cocteau remembers Proust in *La difficulté d'être*.

> Do not expect me to follow Proust on his nocturnal excursions and describe them to you. But you may know that these took place in a cab belonging to Albaret, the husband of Céleste, a night cab truly worthy of Fantômas himself. From these trips, whence he returned at dawn, clutching his fur-lined coat, deathly pale, his eyes dark-circled, a bottle of Evian water protruding from his pocket, his black fringe over his forehead, one of his button boots unbuttoned, his bowler hat in his hand, like the ghost of Sacher Masoch, Proust would bring back figures and calculations which allowed him to build a cathedral in his bedroom and to make wild roses grow there.

Throughout his life, Proust vacillated over the probability of a cure for his asthma, and the suspicion that if he lost his peculiar neurological anxiety, his creative impulse would in some way be impaired. Illness had become the condition for creativity. The breathless, drug-riddled organism through which he lived was preferable to health. Asthma set him apart, and his life was lived in accordance with the idiosyncratic dictates most conducive to his work. He who found 'the microbial sunlight of my chandelier' intolerable, withdrew into a permanent state of artificial night, over which imposed reality rose the brilliant sun of his imagination. In a long correspondence with his friend, Georges de Lauris, Proust touched often on the night and illness, the two constituents that were integrated into the minute bibliographies of his nervous condition. Quoting St John, Proust admonishes himself:

> The night comes when no man can work. I am already halfway into this night, Georges, despite fleeting appearances which mean nothing. But you still have light and will have for many long years, therefore work. Then, when life brings disappointments, there are consolations, for true life is everywhere, not in life itself, nor afterwards, but outside, if a term derived from space can have a meaning in a world freed from that state.

Not only was Proust the victim of the persistently deleterious effects of asthma, and a respiratory system hypersensitive to colds, flu and minute changes of bodily temperature, but he suffered from narcotic poisoning. Reluctant to undergo medical diagnoses (and Proust shared affinities with Rilke in his readiness to entertain illness as a form of mystic revelation), he set about prescribing for himself in the attempt to conciliate an alarming nervous condition. There is something that will forever remain secret about Proust's life, a quality that defies even the most exhaustive biography, which has to do with chemical adjustment. The gravitation inwards, the fascination to live through the unconscious and to excavate an architectonics of psyche kept Proust isolated and apart. Drugs create unsociability, for one's own need cannot readily be shared, and this in turn generates a code of secrecy in the user. 'This frantic race, sleepless in spite of illness, this "race towards death" had changed me so much, I no longer recognized myself in mirrors and people in stations asked whether there was anything I needed. . . . And since then

I've spent all the time trying to recover.'

When we read Proust we enter into the complicity of his life, the complex permutations of his inner states, the private mythology that governed his illness. Towards the end of his life, he was injecting himself often injudiciously with a mixture of Evadine and Kola. The latter comprised a solution of adrenalin and hypophysical extract. He had by this time begun to suffer from vertigo, speech impairment and muscular paralysis in his face. He needed to inject himself with an ampoule of adrenalin before undertaking any physical exertion. Opium, veronal and Dial – Proust like all drug users became confused as to the quantity he had taken each day. His doses were misregulated and his aphasia grew correspondingly more pronounced. His need to write found a cotangential impulse in his need to support the undertaking with drugs. The equation between the two functions is a simple one. The man writing out of his nerves, translating his inner life into poetry, feels a corresponding loss for which the drug appears a substitute. The fear of giving away too much leads to an over-compensation of support. Writing is always terrifying, and Rilke gave voice to a profound inner truth when he wrote 'Every angel is terrible.' Externalizing the archetypal substrata of inner space demands a courage that few possess. The risk in undertaking such a pursuit is insanity. Rimbaud walked away from the conflagration he had lit in his nerves. He underwent ravings, withdrawal symptoms at Roche, and out of his hallucinated visions wrote *Une saison en enfer*. Trakl went out on a cocaine high.

Proust continued writing to the very end. Death visited him in the figure of a woman dressed in black, and once she had entered his consciousness the process was irreversible. It was his individual death. He was frightened by the figure, for it occupied too much space, it was still another intrusion on his breathing. There was all the more reason to go. Proust could not have lived with an intruder. He had lived with figures from his past and the inventions of fiction, and all of these were constellated in mental space. He had the advantage of distance on them. And anyhow his work had taken on the independent life he had wished for it. It had arrived.

What are a man's last memories? They may be totally inconsequential, trivial, delirious, or a coherent lucency that consciousness is expanding in proportion to physical extinction. Where was Proust then? He was still writing, involving himself in the dynamics of retrieval, the morphological unit shaped by the imagination, and perhaps there was this door opening in inner space through which he disappeared, his motion fluent rather than obstructed by deoxygenation.

Where are they now, where were they then, the manically suicidal Georg Trakl and the inner cartographer Marcel Proust? Did they come across each other's names on the great microfiche of the dead? And was it at the lugubriously blue Heartbreak Hotel? There is no longer the chance to correct aberrations in the work. That remains as a posthumous incompletion, a desperate swipe at mortal imperfection. Trakl would have arrived in search of drugs for his habit, and Proust who in 1917 had financed the running of Jupien's male brothel, the Hôtel Marigny, a residence to which he was a frequent nocturnal visitor, was no stranger to hotels. The place is a blue illusion. They'll explore its mirrored rooms for ever. Outside in the street someone is selling smack. It would take a thousand years to reach that pusher.

6

Where does anyone go after withdrawal? You are suddenly disinherited, dispossessed of an unconsciously obsessive need, and the world out there is disarmingly different, as though reality had been temporarily switched to a parallel channel, and only now, when you are clear, are you again making contact with the external world. After any prolonged sojourn in the underworld, after years of a peculiar dialectic with drugs, a cellular programming to benzodiazepines, you are left to go it alone. Most tranquillizer users have been assured by doctors that the drug is harmless and non-addictive, so an element of trust has usually been replaced by an inquisitive paranoia. Having had areas of your sensory life eliminated for years by the desensitizing aspects of the drug, you are immediately suspicious as to not only why you let it happen, but why a doctor was so little informed as to go on prescribing a mind-altering drug for the better part of a decade. And I am reminded in my case that I instigated the initiative to detox, no doctor ever suggested that I should remove myself from the drug, or ever raised the issue of deleterious side-effects and the necessity to withdraw from an alarmingly increasing dependency. I had subjectively to evaluate what the drug was doing to me, and it took the onset of an anxiety breakdown for me to realize that the drug was accelerating the periodicity of my severe panic attacks. I got to the point that whenever I took an Ativan I experienced immediate disquiet, something on the inside was rising against me and generating disturbing flashbacks of imagery. I would lie on the bed in a state of panic, unable to sedate myself with the drug I had used for that purpose for over a decade. My moods would shift from the detached to the inflammatory, and I insulated myself from reality, relying more and more on the imaginative input of my work. Something was wrong and I didn't know how or where to locate it. I encountered the terrified impotence we feel at being unable directly to correct inner functions. I was like somebody who realizes the aircraft is going to crash and is powerless to prevent it from going down. I wanted to run away but there was nowhere left to hide. Spotlights had been turned on in my old underground refuges and I had to get out of the place.

I remember coming home one day, and out of a perverse desire to reassure myself, checking through the extraordinary cache of tablets I had accumulated, many of the boxes already well beyond their expiry date. I found I had in my possession over three thousand tablets, a reserve that would ensure I was screened from every threatening manifestation of reality. I used to think that when death came I would simply increase my intake of the chemical and remain impervious to whatever transitional psychic state dying involved. I would move from one unreality to another without any sense of dislocation. The drug would take away fear of everything. I was a long way out on a pharmaceutical trajectory, the receptor sites in my brain constantly on call for Ativan. If I went down the street to the local off-licence, I checked my jacket pockets to see that they were lined with the drug. I began to think of the shortest journeys in terms of the sense of threat they evoked, and without my properly knowing it the drug was starting to make me agoraphobic, a condition that was to restrict my every movement in the stages of withdrawal. I was becoming apprehensive about travelling in or across London, and began to assess areas by the availability of taxis, for I was already contemplating means of making a quick exit from the street should I be overtaken by panic. I would compulsively check and recheck the safety of my tablets. My hand was closed over them in a weird conspiratorial ritual. And if the flip-out came, I mean if the pavement started travelling the other way and my visual field was upended on the dynamics of a weird spin, the sweat minting itself on my hands, my breathing growing consciously and progressively shallower, red hallucinations starting up with the accompanying fear that I was about to lose my sense of identity, then I would frantically search for a taxi, push down the windows to increase maximum air flow, and crush tablets into my mouth in the hope of allaying the attack. I would be obsessed with the fear of projectile vomiting and of losing consciousness in the taxi. Would I remember my address? Did I know who I was? And had the district in which I lived disappeared? I was being conveyed to a parallel universe.

When the attack grew less constrictive, and the hallucinated images were less up front, then the corresponding sense of euphoric relief was huge; it was like learning to breathe again as the world stabilized and I regained some connective bridge with reality. I began to go out with an emergency bag containing Ativan, Valium, anti-nausea tablets and a small bottle of whisky. These were my resources when it all became too much. It was as if I were carrying around a life-support unit. But I was without any sense of prolonged dysphoria, and with the instinctive phasing-out by which memory associations allow us to disconnect from psychophysical trauma, I lived with the hope that my panic would decrease. On the contrary, the crises accelerated into a breakdown and I developed a sensory intuition that I was being poisoned by the drug, and that until I withdrew I would be the victim of pharmaceutical toxicity. Desperation led me to explore avenues of alternative help, and I benefited greatly from weekly acupuncture sessions, aromatherapy massage to assist with muscular tension, and the adoption of yoga in the Kashmir tradition, which helped me to explore the idea of breath as global sensation rather than as a continuous psychic manipulation. Panic instates shallow breathing, and in turn this is translated into neuromuscular tensions, and by learning to listen to the breath and to feel with the whole body I was able to anticipate severe crises and to modify their devastating intensity.

As the necessity for me to withdraw deepened into a reality, I was introduced to Dr Francis Keaney at the London Institute. Using Valium as a substitute for Ativan, I began the gradual process of substitution, and by replacing one substance with its corresponding equivalent, and then by reducing the latter according to what seemed a metabolically tolerable level, I succeeded over a period of twelve months, and often by using a nail-file on the granular tablet to eliminate the chemical need for benzodiazepines. But the inner adjustment, the psychotic hallucinations, the rehabilitation to life without tranquillizers, the strong residual traces of agoraphobia, sensory changes for touch, noise, vision and smell, feelings of unreality, delusions and paranoia were to persist over a period of another two years.

These symptoms are still easily provoked by periods of overwork and nervous exhaustion. I no longer see blood sweating out of the walls, or hear conflagratory fire raging in the street, or encounter lions sitting at my feet as they did for a whole summer, but I am aware that a rift or flaw has occurred in me, and that I must not injudiciously overload my nervous circuit. Addicts get clear but they remain vulnerable casualties. The fissure will never properly heal, and alcoholism and logotherapy are often the surrogate destinies adopted by damaged addicts. Other users threatened by the temporary psychosis of withdrawal prefer to backtrack and return to the security of the drug. The majority of involuntary addicts will remain on benzodiazepines for the rest of their lives, unless some form of deep emotional crisis precipitates the degree of self-awareness required to detoxify. You can do it the slow, painful way I chose, a method that involves an underworld journey back to the light, or you can elect to have NET, Meg Patterson's black-box treatment, which speeds up the process, but neither method in the case of long-term dependency is unaccompanied by acutely discomforting withdrawal symptoms. Because of development of tolerance to the prescribed dosage, benzodiazepines tend to be ineffectual in lowering anxiety symptoms after a period of six weeks, and yet doctors continue to prescribe them for as many years. All secondary symptoms are construed as primary ones, and so the dosage is increased in proportion to the patient's reported anxiety. This is what it means to be hooked.

Today I was in Wardour Street, and I stepped into the adjoining Peter Street in order to connect with Berwick Street market, when a flashback jumped at me. It was like being physically thrown to the ground, only the collision happened on the inside. The hallucinated phenomenon was an imposingly cyclical obsession that had threatened me psychically during my period of breakdown and withdrawal. The figure of a wounded man representing all the repulsive antitheses to life that I most feared, someone dressed in a shabby black greatcoat, a loser who possessed a formidable insider's knowledge of my most secret fears, materialized out of the crowd, his compulsive magnetism to my psychic energies making him throw me into complete terrified isolation. This man had discovered me again, his gravitation towards my vulnerability left me without defences. He had attached himself to me through some weird form of symbiosis, some intrusive leakage to my interior. The person I had always dreaded becoming, a figure comprising components of my dead father's masculinity and of an outlawed and reviled, ageing queen, was attempting to break back into my awareness. I felt the nausea rise in me, there was a concentrated red aura to the image, my sense of smell was seriously over-alerted, and I had the impression I wanted to run away, run all the way back to childhood and take refuge in a state of non-experiential innocence. I wanted to be back in my particular school yard, the afternoon acquiring a deep-green shade under the apple trees, all time suspended as though my body-clock was not yet in motion. Instead I was undergoing the strange disorientating spin to hallucinatory panic, I was in a cold sweat and anxious to get off the crowded streets.

I returned to Wardour Street, frantically searching for a taxi and attempting to earth myself by deepening my breathing. The hallucinated figure wouldn't go away but kept on returning to my visual field. In the past I would have had immediate recourse to Ativan, and symptomatic vestiges of agoraphobia were amplifying my panic. Like all anxiety victims I thought I was going to die in the street. The solitariness of the individual in a big city was powerfully impressed on me. Nobody would stop, and if they did, it might be for the wrong reasons. I had thought I was clear of residual withdrawal symptoms, but at random, two and a half years later, I was being blown away by hallucinatory terror. It was as though the whole process was being recycled and as if my brain chemistry was still programmed to repeat psychotic incidents. The red terror had returned, and I was hardly seeing at all as I searched through the Soho streets for the reassuring presence of a black cab. There were times during the drug years when I had literally prayed for a taxi's arrival, in those desperate moments of crisis, and here I was repeating it all over again on an ordinary Friday afternoon in busy Soho.

Discomfort, physiologic imbalances, autonomous hallucination, all these factors had returned on some negative reverse spiral, only there was a sense of slight distancing, as though the psychic action were taking place at a more removed space than the direct subjective identification I had experienced in the maelstrom of withdrawal. I had a distinction between subject and object: me and it. In the confused persecution delusions I had undergone in the initial stages of withdrawal I was totally identified with psychic content. I was the autonomous happening, and I watched myself, shirt in flames, roll slowly down a steep gradient towards a bottomless, black lake. All the metaphysically involuted infrastructure of a Poe story becomes a reality in states of advanced terror.

What the addict seeks is exclusion from reality and the occupation of an idealistically enriched imaginative space that runs parallel with other people's lives but at the same time rarely intersects with their criteria for living. In his book *Drugs: Medical, Psychological and Social Facts*, Peter Lawrie astutely observes:

> The addict's whole life is organized to remove any dependence on humanity: given his drugs, he is self-sufficient, able to generate his own satisfactions and guilts and to live a rich emotional life independent of the outside world. He therefore has no motives for communication when things are going well; when he does present himself for treatment it is often not because he wants to be cured of addiction, but because his addiction is not working as it should.

We have encountered this sense of reclusive isolation in Anna Kavan's life-style, and it is a recurring feature in so many addictive sensibilities. The user is travelling in a different direction from the non-user, his gravity is to his own interior, and towards the imaginal rather than the materially realized. The inner journey contradicts the outer, and the opposition between these contraries is a source of constant social and ideological tension. Governments and the collective rationale demand an organized work ethic, one directed towards a healthy economy, and the addict or the inner-orientated are seen to fulfil no role in that regimented function. They are living on another planet, a parallel universe situated in a self-preoccupied mental space. They are the dispossessed who live by imagined resources rather than real values. Addiction is of course synonymous with self-differentiation and the need to individuate independent of familial or social influences. Can I ever be truly myself in a world governed by judicial dictates and socially conformist strictures? The addict dreads being depathologized for fear of losing individual distinction. The drug represents a form of self-projective image. Pharmaceuticals instate a secret marriage with individual chemistry.

One might argue that creativity is inextricably linked to the pathological, and that without the disease we lack the creative principle. It was Jung who pointed to the deification of the pathological: 'The gods have become diseases; Zeus no longer rules Olympus but rather the solar plexus, and produces curious symptoms for the doctor's consulting-room.' Psychopathologies are symptomatic of our awareness of inner events, and suggest the sanctity of madness, and the richly informing agent it is to the imagination. It is a subject of deep consternation to all those who have touched on the inexhaustible properties of the creative imagination to find the arts so often inexpressive of that abundantly fertile source, as though a materialist rationale were the informing agent behind genius rather than the subversively upending dynamics of poetic delirium.

And what of that traumatizing regression I had experienced in Soho? It will of course recur, in the way that hallucinatory phenomena cannot be dissociated from the addictive/breakdown sensibility. Like millions of addicts I am clear, but I shall never be free of pathological symptoms. They are the modified substrata out of which I live and create, and they are a reminder to me to celebrate and intensify the moment before psychic menace returns. If I think back to the years of emotional desensitization, I am lost. I allowed myself unquestioningly to become dominated by a prescribed drug, and to enter into a pact with a doctor who prescribed for me and was the agent behind the chemical policing of my neurology. Almost as if frozen in a slow-motion time-warp, the pact was to continue for over a decade. Neither doctor nor patient made any attempt to break the inexorably complicitous relationship that was centred upon a prescription pad and a dependency. I would freeze into a cold sweat at the idea of the drug's ceasing to exist. To counteract the fear of losing the source, I continued to accumulate. I received quadruple repeat prescriptions, I got the drug from a second doctor, and so my supply increased. I hoarded it like loot; my blue pills were the funeral statuary in a pyramid. Whatever else happened in life, I wasn't going to be disconnected from my supply. I would calculate the number of years I could live on the cache I had buried away. But I still needed more. I would climb a blue mountain of tablets. They would slide beneath my feet like small pebbles. The name Ativan would be flying on the flag topping the summit. Being dependent is a life function, it eats up energy, you fight with the incessant paranoid possibilities of there being an interruption in your supply.

What we all need is a witness. How am I different without the drug, and in what ways have I changed? There is my own subjective reading of the issue, and there is the objective assessment made by friends. Areas have opened up in me that were closed before, there is more space in my emotions and less fear contained in my naturally phobic obsessions. I no longer reach for my blue tablets on waking in the morning, that compulsive first action of the day which became my inveterate habit. There was never a question of my having to remember whether I had taken the drug, and if there were the occasional lapse, my metabolism would alert me within hours. I would reach a panicked zero without it. The period of total de-energization that surrounded withdrawal has largely been rectified, but immediate loss of energy was indicated by even an involuntary break with the drug. It was like attempting to drive a car without fuel, the metabolism churning to a halt.

Letting go of the drug is like attending one's own funeral. Somebody was being buried and that person was me. The initial sense of euphoria attendant on the act is soon dispersed, and the process of readjustment is painfully slow, for the big achievements that came so quickly after the initially painful retreat from the drug were like fast-forwarding, and are later modified by regressive symptoms. It is a matter of not being overly discouraged by recurring symptoms, and of attempting to distance oneself from the anxiety site. Gradual restimulation of the depressed endorphin system will counter craving, anxiety and lethargy, the three predominant symptoms inherent in detoxification, but there is a time-scale involved in this, and the subject may often feel that things will never come right again, and that some vital component has gone missing and will now never be retrieved. We find it so hard to locate a psychic dysfunction. Whatever the particular illness, we feel we lack the means to address the symptoms, and so the questions most often raised are 'Why me?' and 'How can I help myself?'

We are all capable of doing unconscious damage to ourselves. You get addicted and you go on with the habit and life goes on, and when you swing round to face the issue five or ten years have hurried by, and there is no real accounting for why it happened and continued. But the process of disengagement is a long one, and the evaluation of psychological imbalances may begin only then. What was the perverse trajectory I pursued, and where and how would it have ended? I got off before the last stop, but why was I so far down the line? I boarded the train, but others helped me and remained standing on the platform. My particular journey was complicated by an over-active imagination, which together with the disturbance created by drug input generated a syndrome leading to breakdown. If I saw lions crossing the high street, or encountered badly defaced war survivors returning home to nowhere, it was as a part of reintegration, a facing into psychotic phenomena in order to go clear. Everywhere at this moment of writing there are people terrified of going mad, the addicted, those undergoing breakdowns, others living through the amplified panic of withdrawal; there is this huge fear that sanity will never again be reattained, and that severe anxiety and hallucination will become a permanent state.

There are drivers searching the road for the imaginary bodies they believe they have hit, there are the obsessively phobic whose intolerance of all manner of sensory disturbance inhibits an expansive life expression, and many of these people will have taken refuge in psychoactive drugs to compensate for feelings of anxious dysphoria. It is often the latter state which the addict is attempting to feed with pills. I can't name or locate the disquiet but it needs pharmaceutical attention, or at least there is some metabolic change if chemicals are administered. Anti-anxiety drugs when they are first used often cause a high, but over long-term dependency the subject feels little more than an assuaging dialogue with the drug. You need it in order to set up a familiar vocabulary of chemical discourse, but the substance slowly anaesthetizes the emotions, and gradual desensitization, observed not by the subject but by others, takes over. In a withdrawal period that lasted for over two years I was able at times to reconnect with deep emotional states that had previously been kept in cold storage. And what was a reversible psychosis began to recede, interrupted by pathological flashbacks, although the way through is different for everyone, and the severity of symptoms may be mitigated in individuals with a more earthed and practical hold on living. My condition was not helped by the fact that I continued to do imaginative work at times of acute crisis, I persisted in overloading a circuit that was already exhausted and under huge stress, and so the way through the tunnel was slow and excruciatingly painful. The only objective to reach the other side was the memory of pain already encountered, and the need to convert territory gained into a positive acquisition.

There was a clear sense too of journey involved, as though I were moving away fraction by fraction from a disaster area. It was as if there were a fire raging somewhere and I mustn't look back at its cyclonic core. Rather as in the Orphic myth I had to keep my eyes on the god's blue cloak in front, I had to persist in eating up the road ahead no matter the terrifying hallucinations encountered on the way. It was a journey through the underworld, in which night imagery was observed during the day and the oneiric became part of autonomous consciousness rather than being encountered through the unconscious in dream. I seemed to be living on a reverse spiral of psychic confrontation.

Things jumped out at me in the street, in a café, in conversation with a friend, and I was paranoid that someone else might witness my hallucinated encounter. Friends commented on the terror in my eyes but could see no further. I who had made poetic derangement my subject in a string of novels and non-fiction books, found myself still another casualty in that long line of realized breakdowns. And breakdown is self-defining, one feels in a process of inner fragmentation, the pieces don't fit, and the dysfunctional aspects of nervous behaviour are blown up inwardly and magnified out of proportion. Sweat pours out of one's hands and out of the walls. I would listen all day to the ambient strains of Eric Satie's lyrically repetitive piano compositions, finding in those elusive sound-clusters some thread that took me away from immediate suffering. And when the dark dropped I grew terrified of experiencing panic attacks, I grew afraid to sleep in case I was jolted out of that state by tachycardia and the whole subsequent process of hyperventilation. So it persisted. Nightfall was synonymous with crowded fear, and dawn with psychological relief and the notion that help was near at hand. Panic was associated with primal, chthonic influences and the whole underworld repertoire of nocturnal menace. Who would come to assist me in the deep night, what doctor running the length of the street with his black bag would be there at the time of crisis?

I wrote the first half of this book in the agony of withdrawal, hoping in that way not only to monitor an inner dialogue of intense terror but to keep a hold on reality by means of the physical act of writing. I could not do that in solitude, I went out each day to the same café in which I am writing this now, and drew solace from the human company around me. I was at that time invaded by inner and outer terror and the interchange of phenomena contributed greatly to my condition of permanent disquiet. Did I not half expect the dejected and ruined figure of Charles Baudelaire to drag by in chains on the pavement? His life involved such inconsolable despair that it is almost impossible not to project this state on his posthumous being, the drugged poet beaten by the hostility of the bourgeois and tasting his own funeral like grey wedding-cake.

We begin again and again in life from states that we originally conceived as insurmountable in our apprehension of their complexity. The broken love affairs, divorces, the deaths of parents, lovers and friends, all the impossibles that we expect never to outlive we find ourselves having to encounter and go beyond. Addiction too appears unbeatable until some inner dictate asks that we begin the depathologizing process, which is withdrawal. Detoxification and rehabilitation are big events in the series of trauma-metamorphoses we undergo in life. We are forced to change in order to continue, and once we enter into the momentum of the new reality, it is a process in which pain is being transformed into a purposeful future.

What I am left with is the absolute knowledge that I would never voluntarily use benzodiazepines again, but the drug is part of my chemical biography, and its profound influences on my life and work are something I tolerate and accept rather than recriminate against as a negative pathology. How would it have been different without the habit? All addicts ask themselves this question when they get clear. What were the possibilities missed, and were the horizons narrowed by dependency? Would one's work have been different if it had come from an unmediated source? These are hard assessments to make, for one lives and works with what is available, and much of the hallucinated substrata to my writing was there before I began the chemical journey with benzodiazepines and other subsidiary tranquillizers. Seeing for the poet is a form of immediate visual transformation, the universe is changed by the act of image-making, the eye affords access to the universe, but it is the inner eye that photosensitizes the visual exchange between internal and external phenomena. Within that dynamic, or neurologically within a field governed by temporal lobe lability, the implosive constituents of image occur. The vocabulary of the imagination is imagery, a process in itself far removed from the continual attempts by the media to normalize the arts, and to substitute reportage for inner discovery. The normal or the rational make an art out of reaffirming the universe they already know and confirming its uneventful rationale; the imaginative or temporal lobe types attempt to transform the universe into metaphor, and to see it as a base awaiting conversion into the marvellous. Surrealism is the most perfect representation of transferring inner mechanistics to outer, often as a tangible construct pointing to the constellation of images in inner space. Are not Dali's canvases a map of the oneiric continents? And in the need to advance an inner topology, why should we settle for diagrams of the pedestrian?

'The real cure for addiction,' writes Meg Patterson, 'requires revolution – spiritual revolution', and her pioneering work with neuro-electric therapy for addictive disorders is backed with the profound belief in inner change and direction, transformation on the inner plane supplying the qualitative courage to transfer that advance to the external world. Mind-altering substances have become a way of life to generations disillusioned by the materialistic void, and accustomed to the ruthless media invasion of almost all individual privacy. Audio-visuals have stepped into every living space, and the quiet and reflection needed to advance self-awareness and to review inner changes have been under such massive attack that the way out for many has become chemical migration and the secret discourse established by a drug. Denied time and natural retreat into the precincts of inner space, a post-sixties' culture has looked for immediate chemical switch-overs to other worlds, and so the whole ethos of recreational drugs has taken an all too understandable hold on living. It is the quickest way to go somewhere else. You buy your stuff and you are on a journey away from a restrictive material ethos. The latter half of the twentieth century has in the West, as a progressively despiritualized ethos, seen a desperate need to trigger with mind-altering drugs, in other words to get the hell out of a bureaucratically institutionalized system. The invidious system with its microfiche check on all the individual's informational data has over-policed the fundamental human need for secrecy. Over-exposed, we take refuge in subverting the system by going where it can't find us, out on a trip or in the pacifying count-down of opiates. Revolution takes the form of a pharmaceutical spiral, a long arm extending into the recesses of inner space. And isn't the bureaucrat also coking up in retreat from his own intolerable ideology? We blow our minds because we can't bear the rationale we have created. And shouldn't the emphasis be on the process of imagination, the cultivation of the latter so that we find a more celebratory inner route to the future? The bias of political power seems always to rest with the unimaginative, so that a deleterious antagonism to the inner dynamic becomes the prevailing ideological voice. And desensitization of the inner creates the complex socioneurological problems that may create a drug-dependent society.

What is our need? Is it mortality and the temporal linearity by which we live, the fear of insanity, age, illness and death, the apparent terminal obstruction to the fluency of our mental lives which creates this craving for assuagement? In the West we lack a resting-point, there are no stopping-off places in the incessant cycle of doing rather than being. Drugs alter the state in the way that Cocteau took opium in order to get off an express train he imagined was hurtling towards death. Drugs are a jab at perceiving things outside of their correlation with time. We live inside the fertile cosmology of an archetypally constellated inner space, but we are forced all the time to evacuate that cosmos to meet the demands of practical living. Drugs may be a means to finding out what is really going on inside and of reshaping that potential. What is clear is that when physical or emotional damage ensues as a consequence of the drug, clearly the effects are retrograde. Getting burnt or done in minimalizes the drug's vocabulary. The imbalance deteriorates into physical dysfunction.

Ultimately we are still unable at the end of the twentieth century to reverse cellular ageing and circumvent death; we are all still in the process of dying, no matter our hopes for biological and interplanetary migration. Psychoactive drugs play an important role in our lives, and today Prozac has become the big hope for a serotonin-regulated society wishing to level out the down-pockets and the vertical bang into depressed states. It could be that the use of such drugs to counteract the nervous terror instated by serious or terminal illness may be of benefit to a society disquieted by reasons of its mortality.

Post-drugs and post-withdrawal? Autumn again, as Rimbaud wrote, with a sense of resignation to a familiar mood, an inner one in which big red leaves rain in the heart. We go on with our psychic infrastructure, the inner landscape that is part of the topography of psyche. We live with inner film, the images, ideation and recurrent obsessions that characterize the process of individuation, and after withdrawal most of that is still there, only perhaps there is more clear space and a different quality to sensory experience. It is as though light has come through, the way it does quite dramatically after a summer rainstorm, the indigo density of cloud rolling away to blue-blue vistas. There is clearance, and a certain amazement at lack of immediate unspecified dysphoria. It was the unspecified anxiety that had contributed so much to the sense of unmitigated apprehension I had felt on benzodiazepines. The nagging terror of the neutral void in which an irreversible anguish never stops.

I am one of those who never takes a concretized future on trust. I don't even expect my neighbourhood street to be there tomorrow, it could all change like a film-set, the props claptrapping away into the sky, the whole illusory metaphor telescoping to vanishing-point. What I believe in is the power of the imagination as reality, awaking to find the inner has become outer, and that the great cities of the imagination are there for the taking.

Today I was walking down Old Compton Street to meet a friend. No panic, no sudden grab to check if my pockets are loaded with Ativan and Valium, no sudden shortening of my breath, or sudden vertiginous up-ending of perspective, but a near-stability, a feeling of being earthed enough not to be thrown out of orbit. No sweat pouring out of my hands or streaming across my shoulders. I hope it will continue like this. One good day, two, three in a row, a gradual levelling out, association rather than dissociation, and I still notice panic symptoms in others, those who are growing distressed in the crowd, or who are mildly agoraphobic, the old heat as I knew it, and fear of catastrophe. I tell myself the ice won't break, my footing is sure, there is no big rift in the sky, and the ladder waiting for me to climb into the sky is dismantled. The pot of gold is securely in my head.

Autumn again. Living again. Breath as it travels free. There is a world out there that the dependent have to learn to take on trust. Fear is at the root of all addiction, the unspecifiable fear that lives in one like the vague apprehension of getting sprung in a late-night underground car-park. What will jump out of the oily dark, and what will jump out of the psyche? It's a London afternoon. You have to take some time out of writing in order to know what's out there, and how it all feels after drugs. I shall hang around a bit, meet some friends, and continue.

Books Consulted

André Breton, *L'amour fou*. Paris: Gallimard, 1937.

——, *Arcane 17*. Paris: Société Nouvelle des Editions Pauvert, 1944.

David Callard, *The Case of Anna Kavan: A Biography*. Peter Owen, 1992.

Jean Cocteau, *Opium: Journal d'une désintoxication*. First published 1930. Paris: Club Français du Livre, 1957. (*Opium: The Illustrated Diary of his Cure*, trans. by Margaret Crosland, Peter Owen, 1957; rev. paperback edn, 1990.)

——, *La difficulté d'être*. Monaco/Paris: Editions du Rocher, 1947. (*The Difficulty of Being*, trans. by Elizabeth Sprigge. Peter Owen, 1966.)

Frank Graziano (ed.), *Georg Trakl: A Profile*. Carcanet Press, 1984.

Ronald Hayman, *Proust: A Biography*. Heinemann, 1990.

James Hillman, *The Myth of Analysis*. New York: Harper Torchbooks, 1978.

——, *Healing Fictions*. New York: Station Hill Press, 1983.

Jack Hirschmann (ed.), *Artaud Anthology*. San Francisco, Calif.: City Lights, 1965.

C.G. Jung, *Letters*, Vol. 2. Routledge & Kegan Paul, 1976.

Anna Kavan, *Sleep Has His House*. Cassell, 1948; Peter Owen, 1973.

——, *Ice*. Peter Owen, 1967.

——, *Julia and the Bazooka and Other Stories*. Peter Owen, 1970.

Peter Lawrie, *Drugs: Medical, Psychological and Social Facts*. Penguin, 1974.

Henri Michaux, *Misérable miracle*. Monaco/Paris: Editions du Rocher, 1956.

——, *L'infini turbulent*. Paris: Mercure de France, 1957.

Meg Patterson, *Hooked? NET: The New Approach to Drug Cure*. Faber and Faber, 1986.

Octavio Paz, *On Poets and Others*. Carcanet Press, 1987.

Marcel Proust, *Letters to a Friend*, trans. by Alexander and Elizabeth Henderson. Falcon Press, 1949.

——, *Letters to His Mother*, trans. by George D. Painter. Rider, 1956.
——, *Selected Letters*, Vol. 2, 1904–1909, trans. by Terence Kilmartin. Collins, 1992.
Rainer Maria Rilke, *The Notebook of Malte Laurids Brigge*, trans. by Stephen Mitchell. Picador Classics, 1985. (*Die Aufzeichnungen des Malte Laurids Brigge*. 1910.)
Francis Michael Sharp, *The Poet's Madness: A Reading of Georg Trakl*. Ithaca, N.Y.: Cornell University Press, 1981.
John Strausbaugh (ed.), *The Drug User*. New York: Blast Books, 1989.
Unica Zürn, *L'homme-jasmin*, trans. by Ruth Henry. Paris: Gallimard, 1971.

All translations quoted in the narrative are the author's, unless otherwise indicated above. Place of publication of each of the works listed is Great Britain, except as noted.

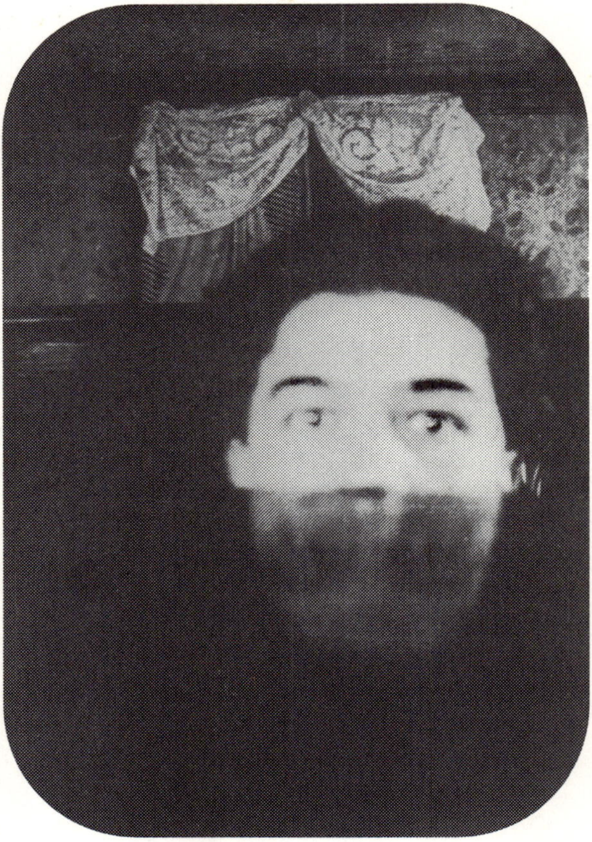

from an image by André Breton – photographer unknown